PANCREATITIS DIET COOKBOOK

150+ Foolproof Delicious Recipes To Reduce Inflammation, Control Pain, and Manage Mild and Chronic Pancreatitis

POLLY DOUGLAS

TABLE OF CONTENTS

INTRODUCTION...12

PANCREAS DISEASES EXPLAINED...14

The Pancreas...14

Endocrine Function...15

Exocrine Function...15

Diseases That Affect The Pancreas...15

UNDERSTANDING PANCREATITIS 17

PANCREATITIS SYMPTOMS & CAUSES.......................................19

Pancreatitis Causes..19

Types of Pancreatitis Causes...20

THE DIAGNOSIS & TREATMENT OF PANCREATITIS...............22

Treatment for Pancreatitis...23

Treatment For Acute Pancreatitis (Mild)..23

WHAT IS PANCREATITIS DIET?..24

FOODS TO EAT & FOOD TO AVOID 26

Foods To Eat..26

Foods to Avoid...27

TIPS ON PANCREATITIS DIET COOKING RECIPES 29

Useful Tips for Pancreatitis Diet...29

Exercise Regularly...29

Drink Plenty of Water..29

SHOPPING LIST..30

Fruits & Vegetables...30

Starches 30

Meat/Protein...30

Fats 30

BREAKFAST PANCREATITIS DIET RECIPES 31

1. Salmon & Cucumber Toast 31

2. Pancakes Wraps 32

3. Cinnamon Glazed Waffle Rolls 33

4. Spinach & Quinoa Muffins 34

5. Overnight Oat Pudding Jar...34

6. Zucchini & Chickpeas Frittata 35

7. Oat Pudding with Chia Seeds...36

8. Quick & Easy Shakshuka 36

9. Scramble Egg Whites Wrap 37

10. Asparagus & Tomato Omelet..37

11. Fluffy Pancakes 38

12. Kale & Quinoa Breakfast Bowl..38

13. Muesli Breakfast Bowl With Berries 39

14. Greek Yogurt with Fig Mulberries Pumpkin Seed 39

15. Sweet Potato Omelet Pie..40

LUNCH PANCREATITIS DIET RECIPES 42

16.   Vegan Baked Navy Beans 42

17.   Hatch Chile "Refried" Beans 43

18.   Indian Butter Chickpeas 44

19.   Mediterranean Quinoa With Pepperoncini 45

20.   Coco-Nutty Brown Rice 46

21.   Herbed Harvest Rice 46

22.   Veggie "Fried" Quinoa 47

23.   Chicken Salad Delight 48

24.   Parsley Burger 48

25.   Seasoned Pork Chops 49

26.   Taco Stuffing 49

27.   Jalapeno Popper Chicken 50

28.   Tuna Au Poivre 51

29.   Fish Stew 51

30.   Grilled Salmon With Fruit And Sesame Vinaigrette 52

BASIC PANCREATITIS DIET RECIPES 54

31.   Minty Melon with Vinegar 54

32.   Mixed Greens Salad with Honeyed Dressing 55

33.   Apricot Salad with Mustardy Dressing 56

34.   Potato Caraway with Lemony Fillet 57

35.   Vinegary Berry with Orange Salad 57

36. Cucumber and Spinach with Chicken Salad 58

37. Lemony Zucchini with Vinegary Salmon 58

38. Carrot Salad with Lemony Cashew Dressing 59

39. Milky Carrot with Oniony Ginger Soup 60

40. Garlicky Broccoli with Cashew Soup 60

41. Squashy Carrot and Celery Soup 61

42. Mixed Greens Soup with Coconut Milk 61

43. Onion Chipotle Soup with Sage 62

44. Pears with Peppered Fennel Soup 62

45. Scallion with Minty Cucumber Salad 63

SAVORY PANCREATITIS DIET RECIPES

SAVORY PANCREATITIS DIET RECIPES 64

46. Beef & Sweet Potato Enchilada Casserole 64

47. Delicious Buckwheat with Mushrooms & Green Onions 65

48. Yummy Chicken and Sweet Potato Stew 66

49. Healthy Fried Brown Rice with Peas & Prawns 66

50. Asparagus Quinoa & Steak Bowl 67

51. Seared Lemon Steak with Vegetables Stir-Fry 68

52. Vegetable Tabbouleh 68

53. Peppered Steak with Cherry Tomatoes 69

54. Grilled Chicken Breast with Non-Fat Yogurt 70

55. Delicious Low Fat Chicken Curry 71

56. Tilapia with Mushroom Sauce 71

57. Ginger Chicken with Veggies 72

58. Hot Lemon Prawns 72

59. Delicious Chicken Tikka Skewers 73

60. Grilled Chicken with Salad Wrap 74

MEAT PANCREATITIS DIET RECIPES 75

61. Pork Egg Roll Soup 75

62. Pork Casserole 76

63. Delicious Pork Roast Baracoa 76

64. Swedish Meatballs & Mushrooms Gravy 77

65. Cherry & Apple Pork 78

66. Paleo Italian Pork 78

67. Corned Pork 79

68. Chipotle Pork Carnitas 79

69. Slow Cooked Pork Tenderloin 81

70. Pork with Carrots & Apples 81

71. Shredded Pork Tacos 82

72. Pork Ragu with Tagliatelle 82

73. Pork with Olives & Feta 83

74. Bone in Ham with Maple-Honey Glaze 84

FISH PANCREATITIS DIET RECIPES 85

75. Scallop and Strawberry Salad 85

76. Halibut with Fruit Salad 86

77. Poached Cod and Leeks 87

78. Cilantro Halibut with Coconut Milk 87

79. Easy Baked Cod 88

80. Herbed Salmon with Onions 89

81. Chinese Salmon 89

82. Spinach and Scallop 89

83. Crab Salad 90

84. Garlic Cod Soup 90

85. Chili Coconut Salmon 91

86. Clams with Olives Mix 92

SOUPS & STEW PANCREATITIS DIET 93

87. Classy Soup with Carrot and Ginger 93

88. Creamy Soup with Broccoli 94

89. Classic Soup with Butternut Squash 94

90. Thai Soup with Potato 95

91. Extraordinary Creamy Green Soup 96

92. Zingy Soup with Ginger, Carrot, and Lime 96

93. Native Asian Soup with Squash and Shitake 97

94. Peppery Soup with Tomato 98

95. Moroccan Inspired Lentil Soup 98

96. Classic Vegetarian Tagine 99

97. Homemade Warm and Chunky Chicken Soup 100

98.   Indian Curried Stew with Lentil and Spinach 101

99.   Soulful Roasted Vegetable Soup 101

100.   Corn Chowder 102

101.   Egg Drop Soup 103

SNACK PANCREATITIS DIET 105

102.   Okra Fries 105

103.   Potato Sticks 106

104.   Zucchini Chips 106

105.   Beet Chips 107

106.   Spinach Chips 107

107.   Sweet & Tangy Seeds Crackers 108

108.   Plantain Chips 108

109.   Quinoa & Seeds Crackers 109

110.   Apple Leather 109

111.   Roasted Cashews 110

112.   Roasted Pumpkin Seeds 110

113.   Spiced Popcorn 111

DESSERT PANCREATITIS DIET RECIPES 112

114.   Café-Style Fudge 112

115.   Coconut and Seed Porridge 113

116.   Pecan and Lime Cheesecake 113

117.   Rum Butter Cookies 114

118. Fluffy Chocolate Chip Cookies 114

119. Chewy Almond Blondies 115

120. Light Greek Cheesecake 115

121. Fluffy Chocolate Crepes 116

122. Crispy Peanut Fudge Squares 116

123. Almond Butter Cookies 117

124. Basic Almond Cupcakes 117

125. Blueberry Cheesecake Bowl 118

SMOOTHIES PANCREATITIS DIET RECIPES 119

126. Cacao Berry Smoothie 119

127. Greek Yogurt Smoothie 120

128. Pineapple Smoothie 120

129. Blueberry Banana Smoothie 121

130. Blueberry Pie Smoothie 121

131. Strawberry Banana Smoothie 122

132. Mango Pineapple Smoothie 122

133. Avocado Smoothie 123

134. Strawberry Smoothie 123

135. Beet Smoothie 124

136. Turmeric Smoothie 124

137. Spinach Smoothie 125

138. Mint Chocolate Chip Smoothie 125

139. Chocolate Protein Smoothie 125

140. Peach Kiwi Green Smoothie 126

STAPLES, SAUCES AND DRESSINGS 127

141. Savory Herbed Quinoa 127

142. Honey-Lime Vinaigrette with Fresh Herbs 128

143. Creamy Avocado Dressing 129

144. Avocado Crema 129

145. Romesco 130

146. Creamy Turmeric Dressing 131

147. Cherry-Peach Chutney with Mint 131

148. Tofu-Basil Sauce 132

149. Creamy Sesame Dressing 132

150. Almond-Hazelnut Milk 133

28-DAY MEAL PLAN 135

CONCLUSION 138

RECIPE INDEX 140

INTRODUCTION

Is there anything that can be done to prevent repeated attacks of acute pancreatitis?

This would depend largely on the cause of pancreatitis in that person in the first place. So, you will need to work along with a medical professional to pinpoint all the causes that could cost an inflammation increase. This is because there are some causes that, once treated, you could prevent other attacks. A good example of this pancreatitis is caused by gallstones in a patient with a lipid issue. If the physician finds that they were caused solely by the medication they use to treat the underlying lipid issue or an excess of alcohol use, they could easily limit the likelihood of another pancreatitis attack by possibly replacing that medication or avoiding alcohol.

If no definite cause can be found, however, prevention becomes a tad tricky.

As the pancreas is one of the most sensitive organs in the body, it can be easily damaged when you consume food or drink that irritates your stomach. When food enters your intestines, it triggers changes in other parts of your body such as the heart, muscles, and lungs. Excess alcohol intake also raises blood pressure that can lead to pancreatitis; further, high blood pressure may also cause some types of pancreatitis. Overweight people who do not exercise enough and do not have a proper diet are prone to develop this disease. Any time you eat high-fat and high-cholesterol food, for example, you are at risk of developing pancreatitis.

There have been studies, at least in adults that looked at different treatment regimens to see if acute or chronic pancreatitis could be less frequent. They analyzed if the pain experienced could be in between attacks or if things like pancreatic enzyme supplementation or antioxidant cocktails could be used. They also explored if following a low-fat diet only was indeed the way to go.

The results confirmed what was already suspected to be true, and that was that following a low-fat diet that is also moderately high in protein can aid in improving the health of the pancreas and, in turn, successfully lessening future pancreatitis attacks in patients of all ages. There haven't been any specific medication that has been proven to fully prevent all attacks, however, it is recommended that you try to incorporate regular exercise into your lifestyle and that you work along with your doctor to come up with possible pain medication and other treatments to reduce or prevent inflammation in the pancreas.

Okay, now that you have gathered a better understanding of what pancreatitis is, and how to go about better caring for your pancreas. Let's dive into our sample meal plan and delicious pancreatitis diet recipes to improve your enzymes and health.

Please note patients with acute pancreatitis are advised to visit the medical professional or emergency department of the hospital as these patients are typically admitted for up to a week and taken off all foods. During this time, their bodies are provided nutrients via IV fluids, and pain killers are supplied to assist with the associated symptoms. After release, most patients generally are allowed to go back to enjoying their usual balanced diet.

PANCREAS DISEASES EXPLAINED

The Pancreas

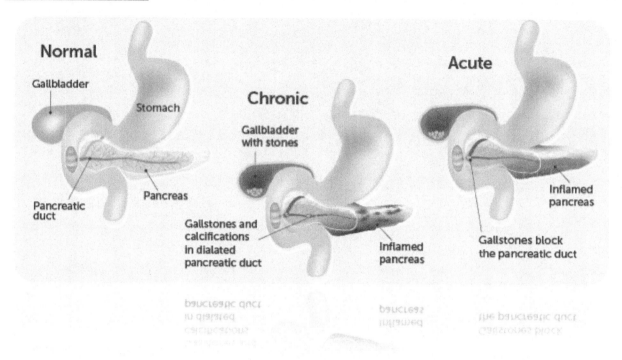

The pancreas is an organ that lies toward the back of your abdomen. It makes digestive enzymes as well as insulin and is key for absorbing many critical nutrients in your diet. There are 2 main functions of the pancreas:

- To aid in digestion (an exocrine function)
- Regulating blood sugar (an endocrine function)

The pancreas can be found behind the stomach and in the upper left of the abdomen. It is surrounded by other organs including your spleen, small intestine, and liver. In terms of texture, the pancreas is spongy. It is between six to ten inches in length and bears the shape of a fish or extended horizontal flat pear.

The pancreas is essentially an accessory digestive plan. It has both exocrine and endocrine functions. The exocrine functions involve the secretion of pancreatic juices from the S&R cells while the endocrine function involves the secretion of glucagon and insulin from the islets of Langerhans. We will see both of them at the histology of the pancreas. It is located posteriorly to the stomach between the duodenum and the spleen with four main parts: the tail, body, neck, and head.

Endocrine Function

The part of the pancreas responsible for the endocrine function is known as the endocrine component and is made of islet cells. These cells secrete two important hormones into your bloodstream and these are glucagon – which is responsible for the increase in blood sugar levels and insulin – which is responsible for lowering blood sugar levels.

Maintaining the proper balance of blood sugar is critical to the proper functioning of vital organs such as the heart, brain, kidneys and liver.

Exocrine Function

The pancreas has exocrine glands that secrete enzymes that play a very important role in the digestive process. These include chymotrypsin and trypsin that help digest protein, lipase that helps in the breakdown of fats and amylase that helps in the breakdown of carbs.

Once food moves from your mouth to your stomach, these enzymes are released into an intricate set of ducts that join the bile duct in the first part of your small intestines (duodenum) which help digest the food.

Diseases That Affect The Pancreas

There are three main diseases that affect the pancreas and these are: pancreatitis, precancerous pancreas conditions and pancreatic cancer. Each of these may present unique symptoms and may require different forms of treatment.

Pancreatitis

This is simply inflammation of the pancreas that occurs as a result of the pancreatic juices accumulating beyond normal levels and beginning to digest the pancreas itself. At onset, pancreatitis manifests as sharp pains that can last for a number r of days before going away. With more progression, pancreatitis may develop into a chronic condition that lasts for years.

Precancerous Pancreas Conditions

Medics and scientists have not been able to establish the exact cause of cancer of the pancreas. What is known is a number of risk factors such as genetic cancer syndromes, cigarette smoking or a family history of pancreatic cancer. There are additional precancerous conditions that also increase the risk of cancer and these are lesions that form on the pancreas such as Pancreatic Intraepithelial Neoplastic (PanIN) AND Intraductal Papillary Mucinous Neoplasms (IPMNs).

Pancreatic Cancer

The most typical type of pancreatic cancer is the Pancreatic Adenocarcinoma which grows on the exocrine glands of the pancreas. Endocrine tumors are not common and only account for less than 5 percent of all pancreatic cancer cases that are reported.

UNDERSTANDING PANCREATITIS

We have so far established that pancreatitis occurs as a result of inflammation that is caused by the pancreatic enzymes starting to digest the pancreas, which should happen.

When you put food in your mouth, a signal is sent to your stomach alerting it that there is food coming through and to thus prepare all the digestive system components. As food goes down your digestive tract, enzymes are released that help in the digestion process. For example, if you eat a delicious piece of steak, the enzymes that are released (chymotrypsin and trypsin) are so potent that they devour the meat very quickly.

Our bodies need these enzymes to be this strong otherwise it wouldn't be possible for you to enjoy a juicy steak or chops. Under normal circumstances, we don't pay much thought to what happens to the food we eat from the moment we put it in our moths to the moment we poop. The truth is that the pancreas plays a pivotal role in the digestive process as it's responsible for the synthesis and release of these enzymes.

When you develop pancreatitis, the secreted enzymes that are normally released into the first part of the small intestine (duodenum), get triggered whilst still in the pancreas. Question is, if these enzymes are actually created in the pancreas, why does the pancreas get hurt? Shouldn't it be able to handle these enzymes?

Well, the above-mentioned process may have oversimplified the process of enzymatic release in relation to digestion. What happens is that these enzymes do not get triggered until they mix with other digestive chemicals, a process that takes place in the duodenum.

However, this does not hold when pancreatitis occurs and the enzymes are actually triggered whilst in the pancreas therein beginning to digest the pancreas. When this happens, we now have a huge problem inside the pancreas. The body being well equipped to stop attack even that which is caused by its own components, activates inflammation.

When pancreatic cells get in contact with the prematurely triggered enzymes, its blood vessel and tissues get inflamed as they are being literally digested and they are trying to 'heal themselves. However, if this persists the self-digestion that the pancreatic tissues and vessels begin to bleed and the pancreas starts to lose function and the enzymes start leaking to other parts of the digestive system, a process that results in a lot of pain.

Pancreatitis on onset has been described as a very sharp and burning pain that is felt right below the ribs or between your abdomen and back. To some, they have described the pain as having thought that they were experiencing a heart attack. Some have fainted while others have had severe bouts of vomiting as a result of pancreatitis.

Pancreatitis can occur as a sudden attack, in some cases it could last for a couple for days while in others it can go for weeks or even months, solely depending on what is the trigger and also the health of the patient in question.

When a person first experiences pancreatitis, there is a chance that this could recur and it is important that they seek medical help in order to determine the cause to make sure it does not happen again.

PANCREATITIS SYMPTOMS & CAUSES

When your pancreas becomes inflamed or begins to break down you will experience discomfort to different degrees with a myriad of symptoms. Some symptoms may disappear without treatment, but severe cases can cause life-threatening complications.

Acute pancreatitis attacks typically happen as a result of gallstones from the gallbladder obstructing the pancreatic duct. The signs to look out for are:

- Abdominal pain
- Nausea
- Fever
- Vomiting

Chronic pancreatitis occurs after repeated bouts of acute inflammation that progressively destroy the gland cells over time. Its symptoms are:

- Greasy and smelly feces
- Unintended weight loss
- Intense abdominal pain
- Nausea and vomiting.

Diarrhea or constipation: this depends on how severe your stomach is hurting. If it hurts a lot, it may cause diarrhea, but if the pain is mild, constipation may occur. This, in turn, causes more stomach pain and cramping.

Sudden weight loss as a result of your body not digesting food properly or you not eating much at all because you feel unwell.

The symptoms of pancreatitis can start out mild and then progress to be extremely painful within 12–24 hours if left untreated. The exact cause of pancreatitis is unclear. This may be the result of infection, virus, wrong enzyme, or a combination of these factors.

Pancreatitis Causes

Pancreatitis is an inflammation of the pancreas, the organ in your body that produces digestive enzymes and helps metabolize food. The most common causes are gall stones, trauma (such as a car accident), and infection (such as pancreatic cancer).

Pancreatitis is a serious illness. The damage caused during an attack can range from mild pain to severe. It may be difficult to diagnose pancreatitis at first because there are many possible causes (i.e., gallstones) that can cause similar symptoms.

Types of Pancreatitis Causes

Trauma

Trauma can be caused by an accident that damages the pancreas or by an injury that causes a direct pancreatectomy. The damage from trauma can often result in severe pancreatitis.

Diabetes

Diabetes is a serious long-term disease that alters how your body deals with the glucose found in your blood. Glucose is a type of sugar that is always present in the human blood. So, when the condition arises, there is always glucose to react to. There are type 1 and type 2 diabetes, but the majority of the people who have diabetes have type 2. In the U.S. alone, around 27 million people live with this condition. Some other 86 million people have prediabetes, a condition just short of diabetes. In this case, their blood glucose is too high to be normal, but also too low to be fully diabetic yet.

Part of the job of your pancreas is to produce a hormone known as insulin. This insulin is the hormone that allows your cells to be able to convert the glucose found in your food into energy. People who live with type 2 diabetes still produce insulin. However, the changes in the cells have made them unable to fully utilize it as they normally should. This is what doctors call insulin resistance.

At the initial stage, the pancreas frantically tries to produce more insulin to compensate for the shortage of glucose in the cells. At a point, the work overload couldn't be maintained. This is when the sugar starts accumulating in your blood instead.

Pancreatic Cancer

Pancreatic cancer, simply put, is the presence of one or more cancerous masses or tumors that develop within the cells of the pancreas. Pancreatic cancer is a disease that rarely occurs. Pancreatic cancer is most common among older men who have heavy drinking habits and smoking. However, pancreatic cancer can also be caused by certain types of cancers (such as lymphoma) or through certain types of radiation therapy.

Infection

Pancreatitis can be treated in many different ways both medically and surgically. There is no cure for chronic pancreatitis but it can be controlled with medication and/or surgery. Even with chronic pancreatitis, the person will not necessarily die from the condition as long as they have access to medical treatment that helps control the symptoms.

THE DIAGNOSIS & TREATMENT OF PANCREATITIS

When a health care practitioner notices symptoms that are consistent with pancreatitis, they will ask the person questions about their symptoms, lifestyle, and habits, as well as their medical and surgical history.

To rule out specific illnesses, health care providers will look to see if the responses to these questions correlate with the findings from the physical examination.

In nearly all circumstances, a laboratory test is required. The body systems listed below are put to the test during the tests:

- The liver, pancreas, and kidney all contribute to these functions (such as pancreatic enzyme amylase and lipase)
- It may indicate infection if you have a fever or are exhausted.
- impaired blood cell numbers due to anemia
- home pregnancy test
- Electrolytes, electrolyte levels, and calcium levels indicate dehydration.

When there are digestive enzymes and insulin produced by the pancreas, blood testing may show equivocal results. Gallstones may be found with imaging testing when it is thought that you have pancreatitis.

Imaging tests listed below may be used for the detection of a tumor.

1. Discomfort caused by pancreatitis, as well as other reasons, maybe identified by X-rays. A chest X-ray may be required.
2. X-ray films are comparable to CT scans in their utility, while CT scans are capable of obtaining greater detail. The CT scan gives a more thorough look into the pancreas and pancreatitis complications, and it yields an image superior to an X-ray picture. The pancreas seems damaged or destroyed during a CT scan. Some doctors suggest getting an MRI.
3. Ultrasounds are a powerful imaging test for determining if the gallbladder, ducts that connect the gallbladder, liver, and pancreas to the small intestine, and ducts that connect the pancreas to the bile ducts and the liver are working correctly.
4. The procedure utilized to assess the pancreas and adjacent tissues during endoscopic retrograde cholangiopancreatography is done under local anesthesia (ERCP).

Treatment for Pancreatitis

The treatments for pancreatitis include measures that assist the patient and the patient's condition depends on the degree of severity. However, as a general rule, morphine is a good pain reliever. To yet, no scientific studies have found that morphine increases the risk of pancreatitis or cholecystitis.

In the case of mild or moderate pancreatitis, the therapy will differ based on whether or not there are complications.

Treatment For Acute Pancreatitis (Mild)

In the treatment of mild acute pancreatitis, admission to a general hospital ward is effective. Up until now, it was believed that it was inappropriate to feed a patient until the inflammation had decreased, but recent research suggests that early feeding is safe and beneficial, and can shorten the time that patients stay in the hospital.

To help with pancreatitis-related lung problems, patients with this condition may have breathing tubes inserted to their noses to provide them with supplemental oxygen. If the patient looks to be improving, the tubes can be removed after a day or two.

To prevent dehydration, fluids will be administered intravenously. Many kinds of pain are alleviated by the use of opioids. In the event of gallstone-induced pancreatitis, early gallbladder removal appears to help the situation.

WHAT IS PANCREATITIS DIET?

The diet for acute pancreatitis varies considerably based on the severity of the disease. In the most severe forms, it is better to avoid any form of oral feeding, both based on food and based on parenteral solutions (nasogastric tube).

This is necessary to keep the organ at rest which, in most cases, is unable to perform its endocrine function or its exocrine function adequately.

Nutrition for severe acute pancreatitis mainly occurs intravenously and is often associated with drugs of the type: analgesic, antibiotic, hormonal (insulin), etc.

The requirements of parenteral nutrition for severe acute pancreatitis are:

- High water content
- Concentration of carbohydrates proportional to glycaemia
- Low lipid content, mainly composed of medium-chain fatty acids
- Medium portion of essential amino acids
- Salts and vitamins in normal quantities.

In the milder forms, however, when the resolution is estimated in approximately 24 or 48 hours, it is possible to forego the intravenous nutritional administration by limiting the water compensation; in some cases, it is possible to start the food-based diet early.

For both situations, when the pancreatic enzyme levels are within the ordinary, it is possible to start with a solid diet.

The basic requirements of this diet are:

- TOTAL elimination of alcohol (including wine with meals) and drinks with other nerves (coffee, tea, energy, etc.)
- High splitting of total energy, with at least 6 small meals
- High water content
- High carbohydrate content, especially with a low glycemic-insulin index
- Low concentration of carbohydrates with a high glycemic-insulin index (especially in the case of diabetes mellitus)
- Low lipid content
- Modest protein content of animal origin, to be progressively increased.

Pancreatitis is a serious digestive disorder that can affect people of any age. It occurs when your pancreas becomes irritated and swollen due to a blockage in bile ducts. In some cases, the pancreas becomes enlarged and filled with little amounts of fluid, while in others it remains hard and shrunken.

Although pancreatitis is a potentially life-threatening condition, most patients with this condition have a good prognosis with appropriate treatment. The goals of treatment for pancreatitis are to reduce pain and inflammation, as well as to support the patient's nutritional needs as they recover from pancreatitis. Diet plays a crucial role in helping patients recover from pancreatitis.

Diet plays a vital role in the health of your gut. When you eat foods that are processed and contain ingredients that aren't natural to your body, you're basically putting poison into your system. Your body then begins to attack itself to rid itself of these toxins, which is why people with chronic conditions, such as pancreatitis, experience flare-ups or attacks.

One of the most important things in life is to take care of your health. Take care of your body and you can prevent many diseases, sicknesses and avoid premature aging. A lot of people are so concerned about what they look like that they forget that it is necessary to look good from the inside.

FOODS TO EAT & FOOD TO AVOID

Foods To Eat

Pumpkin: The pumpkin is rich in vitamin C, potassium, and beta-carotene. It also has low-fat content. In addition, this wild plant also contains a type of fiber that is good for the digestive system. Consuming pumpkin seeds can be an effective way to aid the healing process of pancreatitis because they are a potent antioxidant and contain some calcium, iron, and protein.

Artichokes: These are rich in fiber and calcium with only 2% calories from fat! Consuming artichoke every day can help you overcome constipation issues as well as your pain from pancreatitis since they contain an acid that acts like stomach acid to help you digest food more effectively. Artichokes also contain antioxidants that help with healing and protect the digestive tract.

Raspberries: These are rich in manganese and antioxidants that can help prevent pancreatitis from occurring again. Consuming raspberries regularly can help to protect the body against future inflammation of the pancreas, thus slowing down the progression of pancreatitis.

Herring: It contains a form of omega-3 fatty acids, so eating herring in moderation can help to lower triglycerides by reducing inflammation of the pancreas. Herring also contains calcium and magnesium which can support healthy blood pressure levels.

Quinoa: Consuming quinoa can help improve digestion and prevent constipation due to its complex carbohydrates. You can digest it easily since it is not too high in fiber content but it has adequate amounts of protein.

Sweet potatoes: These are a good source of fiber and nutrients that can help manage constipation. They have vitamin C and beta carotene, both of which help prevent pancreatitis.

Chicken: This is a good source of protein, but you should be careful with it. Some people with pancreatitis have difficulty digesting meats and poultry because their stomach acids may be overly concentrated, due to inflammation of the pancreas. Try not to eat chicken for the first two weeks, and then start incorporating it slowly into your diet after two weeks if no problems arise. Remember to remove any skin from your chicken to avoid excess fat content in your diet during the recovery process.

Figs: These succulent fruits contain a high amount of omega-3 fatty acids, antioxidants, and calcium. Consuming figs regularly can help to increase the levels of good cholesterol while reducing your triglyceride levels.

Sweet corn: This type of vegetable is often overlooked because people do not know what part they should be eating to reap its benefits for their overall well-being. The pods contain a large number of antioxidants, B vitamins, and fiber that help to manage constipation.

Cherries: These juicy fruits are rich in calcium and potassium, as well as other nutrients like vitamin C and beta carotene. Consuming cherries regularly can improve blood pressure levels, thus lowering your risk of developing pancreatitis again in the future.

Foods to Avoid

Foods that contain wheat: This is an ingredient that's used in a lot of bread and pastries and other products, and you shouldn't eat these types of foods unless they're made with gluten-free flour. But even then, it's pretty much impossible to avoid gluten altogether. A better option is to keep your intake low; just do your best not to consume more than 20 grams of wheat per day.

Foods that are known irritants: While it's normal to have a little inflammation in the body after you've had pancreatitis, it's not healthy for long-term exposure to irritants. This is why you should avoid spicy foods or other types of food that could cause burning or discomfort in the digestive tract.

Greasy or fatty foods: Since your pancreas already has problems producing enzymes, this is the last thing you want on top of everything else! You should try to eat foods that are low in fat and only use olive oil, as it's a healthier type of oil than canola oil or soybean oil.

Foods that can cause excessive acid production: The pancreatic enzymes that your body is not producing probably don't need to be supplemented with, as it's not like your system won't produce enzymes on its own. But what you should do is avoid foods that are heavy in acid; for example, stay away from tomato products and citrus fruits.

Foods that have high-fat content: This includes both animal fat and vegetable oils and other chemically-produced fats. Too much fat will cause the liver to produce more bile, which means more work for your pancreas so you can actually digest fatty food! Instead, try eating more complex carbohydrates like whole grains or potatoes, or even beans.

Spicy foods: Believe it or not, spicy foods are considered one of the things you should avoid if you have pancreatitis–so much. Some doctors recommend that their patients avoid any type of spice for 6–8 weeks after they're diagnosed with the condition.

Foods that can cause nausea: This is a common symptom of pancreatitis, and several foods can cause nausea if you eat them. Any food that's known to make you feel nauseous without causing actual vomiting should be avoided; this would include coffee, chocolate, and peanut butter.

Foods with high sugar content: Foods that have high sugar content should be avoided, and this means that you should avoid any sugary snacks or desserts.

TIPS ON PANCREATITIS DIET COOKING RECIPES

Useful Tips for Pancreatitis Diet

- Avoid drinking alcohol
- Ensure you get the recommended dosage of water or electrolyte beverages daily
- Consult your physician about the required supplements or vitamins to assist the decreased functionalities of the pancreas
- Quit smoking, if you are a smoker
- Switch your diet to one that is moderately high in protein, and low in fat that won't further inflame or damage your pancreas

Exercise Regularly

Exercising cannot be compromised in any form for the complete treatment of pancreatitis. 30-minute moderate exercise for at least 30 minutes each day will be beneficial in keeping off risks of developing pancreatitis.

Drink Plenty of Water

It has been rightly said that water is a wonder drug. It is the best medicine for the human body, so one should make sure to have plenty of it. When the patient is treated for pancreatitis, it is important to maintain proper fluid levels in the body. Proper fluid levels will aid digestion and smooth removal of excreta from the body. There should also be enough water in the body to ensure proper absorption of nutrients in the body. Approximately 8 glasses of water a day keeps a person hydrated all day long.

Hence, we have seen that different lifestyle changes will ascertain a person's well-being against pancreatitis disease. People must be proactive and forward in adopting these changes and must not show ignorant behavior during recovery. Such ignorance on the part of the patient can further impair the situation, hence making it difficult to bring it under proper medical control.

SHOPPING LIST

Fruits & Vegetables

Apple

Blueberries

Raspberries

Orange

Banana

Spinach

Cauliflower

Broccoli

Tomato

Green Beans

Starches

Potato

Sweet Potato

Brown rice

Whole wheat bread

Whole wheat pasta

Black beans

Oatmeal

Corn

Meat/Protein

Skinless chicken breast

Skinless turkey breast

Fish

Egg whites

Whole eggs

Tofu

Protein powder

Fats

Olive oil

MCT oil

Almonds

Cashews

Peanuts

Walnuts

Seeds

Low-Fat cottage cheese

BREAKFAST PANCREATITIS DIET RECIPES

1. Salmon & Cucumber Toast

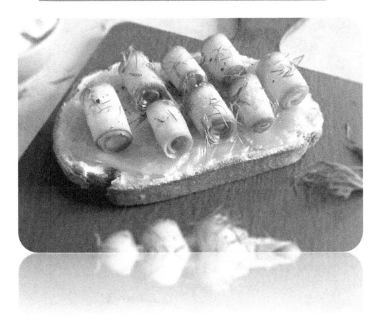

Preparation time: 5 minutes
Cooking time: 5 minutes
Servings: 2
INGREDIENTS:
- 2 slices of whole grain bread
- 2 oz. Greek yogurt
- Salt & Pepper
- 1/4 red onion thinly sliced
- 4 oz. smoked salmon
- 1 cucumber, sliced

DIRECTIONS:
1. Grill bread slice on an electric grill or warm it on griddle. Spread Greek Yogurt on one side of the bread slice
2. Lay smoked salmon, cucumber and onion slice on bread slice. Drizzle salt and pepper on top. Serve and enjoy!

NUTRITION: Calories 222Protein 20 g Carbohydrate 21 g Fats 5 g

2. Pancakes Wraps

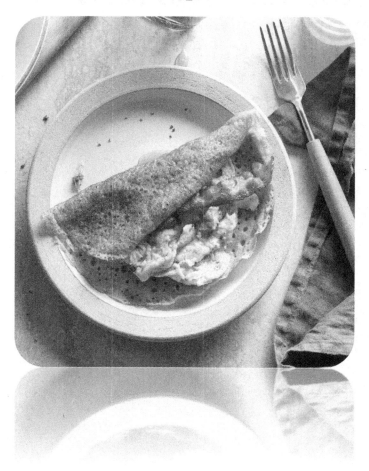

Preparation time: 5 minutes
Cooking time: 10 minutes
Servings: 6

INGREDIENTS:

- 1 1/4 cup spelt flour
- 1/4 tsp. salt
- ¼ tsp. baking powder
- 6 eggs
- 1 cup almond milk
- 1 banana sliced
- chocolate syrup
- 2 oz. Greek yogurt

DIRECTIONS:

1. Mix flour, salt, baking powder in a bowl. Beat eggs with milk in a separate bowl until smooth. Add egg and milk mixture to flour mixture and mix well.

2. Heat griddle over medium heat, spray with non-stick cooking spray and pour ¼ cup of pancakes batter in the middle of a griddle and spread it.
3. Cook pancake for 2-3 minutes each side until the bubbles on top burst and create small holes. Once cooked remove from griddle.
4. Spread low fat Greek yogurt over the pancake and fold it. Top with banana slice and chocolate syrup.

NUTRITION: Calories 226 Protein 13 g Carbohydrate 27 g Fats 8 g

3. Cinnamon Glazed Waffle Rolls

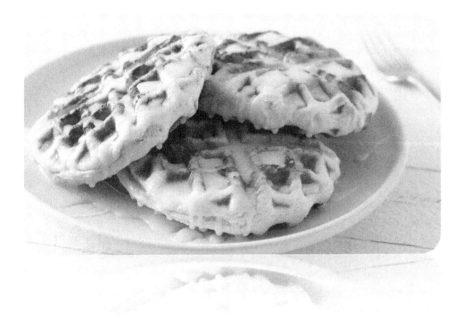

Preparation time: 5 minutes
Cooking time: 10 minutes
Servings: 2
INGREDIENTS:
- 4 eggs
- 1/2 cup oat flour
- 1 tsp cinnamon

Cinnamon roll glaze:
- 2 tbsps. Greek yogurt
- 1 tsp. cinnamon
- 1/2 banana

DIRECTIONS:
1. Switch on the round waffle maker and let it warm. Mix together all waffle ingredients in a bowl. Grease waffle maker with nonstick cooking spray.
2. Pour the waffle batter in a greased waffle maker. Close the waffle maker and cook waffles for about 3-4 minutes.

3. Once waffles are cooked remove from the waffle maker. Mix together glaze ingredients in a bowl. Spread the glaze over waffles and roll-up. Serve and enjoy!

NUTRITION: Calories 237 Protein 14 g Carbohydrate 19 g Fats 10 g

4. Spinach & Quinoa Muffins

Preparation time: 20 minutes
Cooking time: 20 minutes
Servings: 8

INGREDIENTS:
- 2 cups spinach finely chopped
- 1 tbsps. oregano
- 8 eggs
- 1 cup cooked quinoa
- 1 cup buckwheat flour
- ¼ cup almond milk
- 1 tsp. baking powder
- 1/4 tsp. salt

DIRECTIONS:
1. Pre-heat oven to 350 degrees. Beat eggs in a bowl with milk and oregano. Add rest of the ingredients in eggs mixture and mix well.
2. Pour muffins batter in greased muffin tins and bake in the oven for about 15-20 minutes, or until light golden brown.
3. Once muffins are cooked remove from oven. Serve and enjoy!

NUTRITION: Calories 154 Protein 9 Carbohydrate 17 g Fats 5 g

5. Overnight Oat Pudding Jar

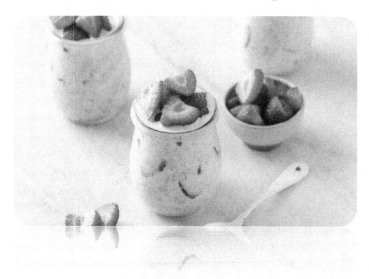

Preparation time: 10 minutes
Cooking time: 0 minutes
Servings: 2
INGREDIENTS:
- banana
- 3/4 cup almond milk
- Pinch sea salt
- 1 cup rolled oats
- 1 1/2 tbsps. chia seeds
- 1 cup strawberries sliced

DIRECTIONS:
1. Add the banana, almond milk, and sea salt in a blender and blend until mixture is smooth.
2. Place the oats and chia seeds in a glass jar and pour the mixture over it and mix well. Cover and refrigerate overnight.
3. In the morning, mix again and add some more almond milk if required. Serve with fresh strawberries slice on top and enjoy.

NUTRITION: Calories 233 Protein 10 g Carbohydrate 51 g Fats 7 g

6. Zucchini & Chickpeas Frittata

Preparation time: 10 minutes
Cooking time: 20 minutes
Servings: 4
INGREDIENTS:
- 1 cup almond milk
- 1 cup chickpeas flour
- 1 tsp. dried oregano
- salt and pepper, to taste
- 4 -6 baby zucchini
- 1 tsp. baking powder
- 4-5 zucchini flowers
- ½ cup thinly sliced red onion

DIRECTIONS
1. Grease non pan over medium heat. Add onion in greased pan and cook for 2-3 minutes. Add zucchini in bowl.
2. Mix chickpeas with milk, baking powder, salt, pepper, and oregano in bowl. Pour this batter over zucchini and onion, top with zucchini flowers.
3. Bake frittata in preheated oven for about 20-30 minutes until cooked through. Serve hot and enjoy!

NUTRITION: Calories 177 Protein 9 g Carbohydrate 24 g Fats 5 g

7. Oat Pudding with Chia Seeds

Preparation time: 10 minutes
Cooking time: 0 minutes
Servings: 2

INGREDIENTS:
- 1/2 cup Oats rolled oats
- 1 tbsp. chia seeds
- 1 cup almond milk
- pinch of salt
- 1 cup strawberries
- yogurt for topping
- berries for topping
- walnuts for topping

DIRECTIONS:
1. Place the oats, seeds, milk, salt, dates in a glass jar with a lid. Place jar refrigerate overnight.
2. Place strawberries on the wall of the serving jar and pour oats mixture in it. Top with oats, strawberries, and chopped walnuts. Serve and enjoy!

NUTRITION: Calories 122 Protein 6 g Carbohydrate 22 g Fats 5 g

8. Quick & Easy Shakshuka

Preparation time: 10 minutes
Cooking time: 20 minutes
Servings: 2

INGREDIENTS:
- 1 onion finely sliced
- 2 red bell peppers finely sliced
- 2 cups tomatoes, chopped
- 1 tsp. spicy harissa
- 4 eggs
- 1 tbsp. chopped parsley
- Salt and pepper to taste

DIRECTIONS:
1. Greased cooking pan with nonstick cooking spray add onions and peppers and cook for 4-5 minutes until soft. Add tomatoes and harissa in pan and cook for another 3-4 minutes
2. Drizzle salt and pepper on top and mix well. Cracks eggs over tomatoes. Cover and cook pan with lid until the egg whites are just set.
3. Drizzle fresh parsley on top and serve immediately with whole grain bread slice. Enjoy.

NUTRITION: Calories 182 Protein 13 g Carbohydrate 13 g Fats 8 g

9. Scramble Egg Whites Wrap

Preparation time: 5 minutes
Cooking time:15 minutes
Servings: 2

INGREDIENTS:

- 1 cup eggs whites, cooked, scrambled
- 1 cup hummus
- ½ cup sweet corn, boiled
- salt and pepper to taste
- 2 homemade corn tortillas

DIRECTIONS:

1. Grease nonstick cooking pan over medium heat, add egg whites with salt and pepper and cook for 2-3 minutes.
2. Spread and divide scramble eggs on each tortilla. Top with hummus and corn.
3. Fold the tortilla and grill for 2-3 minutes and warm up on heated griddle. Slice and serve immediately. Enjoy!

NUTRITION: Calories 365 Protein 21 g Carbohydrate 51 g Fats 8 g

10. Asparagus & Tomato Omelet

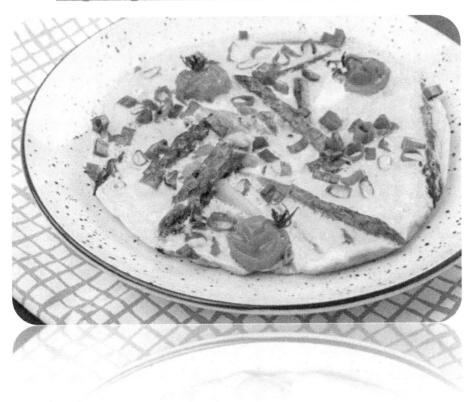

Preparation time: 5 minutes
Cooking time:15 minutes
Servings: 2

INGREDIENTS:

- salt & black pepper to taste
- 4 large eggs
- 5 -6 stalks asparagus, trimmed
- 2-3 tomatoes
- Chopped parsley for topping
- Chopped scallion for topping

DIRECTIONS:

1. Heat oil in a nonstick pan over medium heat. Once the pan is hot, add asparagus and cook for about 2-4 minutes. until asparagus is soft and dark green in color.
2. Beat eggs with salt and pepper in a bowl and pour over asparagus. Cover and cook for about 4-5 minutes until eggs are cooked.
3. Sprinkle parsley, tomato, and scallion on top. Serve and enjoy.

NUTRITION: Calories 193 Protein 15 g Carbohydrate 11 g Fats 10 g

11. Fluffy Pancakes

Preparation time: 10 minutes
Cooking time: 15 minutes
Servings: 2

INGREDIENTS:

- 1 cup oat flour
- 4 large eggs
- 1 tsp. baking powder

Topping:

- coconut cream for topping
- cashew nuts for topping
- strawberry puree for topping

DIRECTIONS:

1. Mix all pancakes ingredients in a bowl until mixture is smooth and fluffy. Heat skillet over medium heat and grease with cooking spray.
2. Pour ¼ cup pancake batter in greased pan and slightly spread it. Flip and cook pancakes for 2-3 minutes per side until slightly brown.
3. Once cooked remove from pan, serve with coconut cream, cashew nuts, and strawberry jam on top. Enjoy!

NUTRITION: Calories 373 Protein 21 g Carbohydrate 36 g Fats 15 g

12. Kale & Quinoa Breakfast Bowl

Preparation time: 10 minutes

Cooking time: 15 minutes
Servings: 2
INGREDIENTS:

- 1 tsp. onion powder
- ½ tsp. salt
- ½ tsp. pepper
- 1 bag baby kale
- 1 cup chickpeas boiled
- 1 cup cooked quinoa
- 1 carrot, sliced and steamed
- 1 tsp. sesame seeds

DIRECTIONS:

1. Mix carrots, quinoa, and chickpeas in a bowl. Mix onion powder, salt, pepper, and oil in another bowl and pour over chickpeas bowl.
2. Drizzle sesame seeds on top. Serve with kale and enjoy it!

NUTRITION: Calories 224 Protein 10 g Carbohydrate 38 g Fats 4 g

13. Muesli Breakfast Bowl With Berries

Preparation time: 10 minutes
Cooking time: 0 minutes
Servings:2
INGREDIENTS:

- 1 cup muesli
- 2/3 cup almond milk
- 1/4 cup blueberries
- 1 apple sliced with skin
- 1 oz. roasted pumpkin seeds

DIRECTIONS:

1. Add muesli with milk in a medium-sized bowl until soft and tendered.
2. Serve soft muesli with an apple slice, blueberries, pumpkin seeds or any other fruit. Enjoy!

NUTRITION: Calories 320 Protein 14 g, Carbohydrate 57 g, Fats 13 g

14. Greek Yogurt with Fig Mulberries Pumpkin Seed

Preparation time: 10 minutes
Cooking time: 0 minutes
Servings: 2
INGREDIENTS:

- 8 oz. fresh figs, halved
- 1 cup low fat Greek yogurt
- 1 oz. pumpkin seeds

- 2 oz. mulberries

DIRECTIONS:

1. Pour low fat Greek yogurt equally in 2 serving jars.
2. Arrange mulberries, pumpkin seeds, and fresh fig slice on top of jar.
3. Serve in breakfast and enjoy it!

NUTRITION: Calories 351 Protein 17 g Carbohydrate 58 g Fats 7 g

15. Sweet Potato Omelet Pie

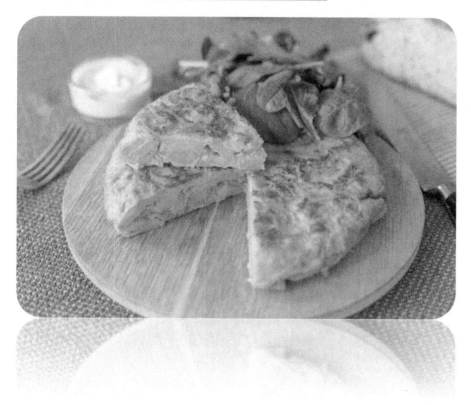

Preparation time: 10 minutes
Cooking time: 20 minutes
Servings: 6

INGREDIENTS:

- 2 sweet potatoes, peeled and sliced into ¼ inch rounds
- 1 onion, sliced
- 10 eggs
- salt and pepper, to taste

DIRECTIONS:

1. Grease ovenproof cast-iron skillet over medium heat. Add sliced potatoes and cook for 8-10 minutes with some water until potatoes are cooked.
2. Add onions and season with salt and pepper. Beat eggs with salt and pepper in bowl.

3. Pour beaten egg mixture over potatoes and cook covered for 5-8 minutes until eggs are set or you can bake it in preheated oven for 20 minutes until egg are cooked.
4. Once brown remove from oven. Serve hot and enjoy!

NUTRITION: Calories 146 Protein 10 g Carbohydrate 10 g Fats 7 g

16. Vegan Baked Navy Beans

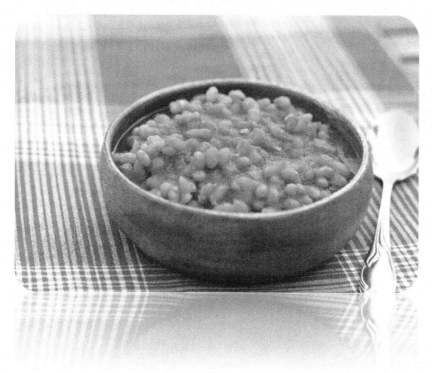

Preparation time: 15 minutes, plus 8 hours to soak
Cooking time: 7 to 8 hours on low
Serving: 4–6

INGREDIENTS:

- 2 cups dried navy beans, soaked in water overnight, drained, and rinsed
- 6 cups vegetable broth
- ¼ cups dried cranberries
- 1 medium sweet onion, diced
- ½ cups all-natural ketchup (choose the one with the lowest amount of sugar)
- 3 tbsp. extra-virgin olive oil
- 2 tbsp. maple syrup
- 2 tbsp. molasses
- 1 tbsp. apple cider vinegar
- 1 tsp. Dijon mustard
- 1 tsp. sea salt
- ½ tsp. garlic powder

DIRECTIONS:

1. In your slow cooker, combine the beans, broth, cranberries, onion, ketchup, olive oil, maple syrup, molasses, vinegar, mustard, salt, and garlic powder.
2. Cover the cooker and set to low. Cook for 7 to 8 hours and serve.

NUTRITION: Calories: 423 Fat: 11 g.Carbs: 78 g.Protein: 16 g.

17. Hatch Chile "Refried" Beans

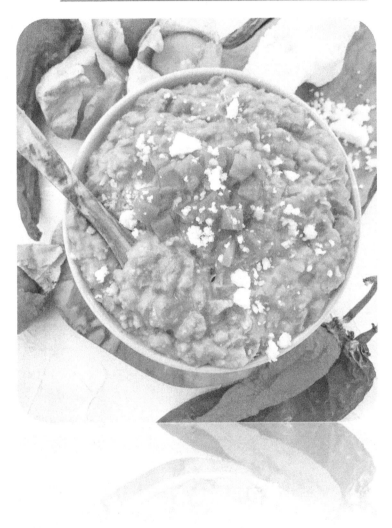

Preparation time: 15 minutes, plus 8 hours to soak
Cooking time: 6 to 8 hours on low
Serving: 4–6

INGREDIENTS:

- 2 cups dried pinto beans, soaked in water overnight, drained, and rinsed
- 7 cups vegetable broth
- ½ medium onion, minced

- 1 (4-ounce) can Hatch green chilies
- 1 tsp. freshly squeezed lime juice
- ½ tsp. ground cumin
- ½ tsp. garlic powder
- ½ tsp. sea salt

DIRECTIONS:

1. In your slow cooker, combine the beans, broth, onion, chilies, lime juice, cumin, garlic powder, and salt.
2. Cover the cooker and set to low. Cook for 6 to 8 hours, until the beans are soft.
3. Using an immersion blender, mash the beans to your desired consistency before serving. If you don't own an immersion blender, mash the beans by hand with a fork or a potato masher.

NUTRITION: Calories: 218 Fat: 0 g.Carbs: 49 g.Protein: 16 g.

18. Indian Butter Chickpeas

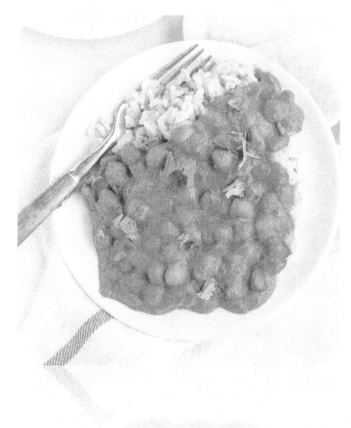

Preparation time: 15 minutes, plus 8 hours to soak
Cooking time: 6 to 8 hours on low
Serving: 4–6

INGREDIENTS:

- 1 tbsp. coconut oil
- 1 medium onion, diced
- 1-pound dried chickpeas, soaked in water overnight, drained, and rinsed
- 2 cups full-fat coconut milk
- 1 (14.5-ounce) can crushed tomatoes
- 2 tbsp. almond butter
- 2 tbsp. curry powder
- 1½ tsp. garlic powder
- 1 tsp. ground ginger
- ½ tsp. sea salt
- ½ tsp. ground cumin
- ½ tsp. chili powder

DIRECTION:

1. Coat the slow cooker with coconut oil. Layer the onion along the bottom of the slow cooker.
2. Add the chickpeas, coconut milk, tomatoes, almond butter, curry powder, garlic powder, ginger, salt, cumin, and chili powder. Gently stir to ensure the spices are mixed into the liquid.
3. Cover the cooker and set to low. Cook for 6 to 8 hours, until the chickpeas are soft, and serve.

NUTRITION: Calories: 720 Fat: 30 g. Carbs: 86 g. Protein: 27 g.

19. Mediterranean Quinoa With Pepperoncini

Preparation time: 15 minutes or fewer
Cooking time: 6 to 8 hours on low
Serving: 4–6

INGREDIENTS:

- 1½ cup quinoa, rinsed well
- 3 cups vegetable broth
- ½ tsp. sea salt
- ½ tsp. garlic powder
- ¼ tsp. dried oregano
- ¼ tsp. dried basil leaves
- Freshly ground black pepper
- 3 cups arugula
- ½ cup diced tomatoes
- 1/3 cup sliced pepperoncini
- ¼ cup freshly squeezed lemon juice
- 3 tbsp. extra-virgin olive oil

DIRECTION:

1. In your slow cooker, combine the quinoa, broth, salt, garlic powder, oregano, and basil, and season with pepper. Cover the cooker and set to low. Cook for 6 to 8 hours.
2. In a large bowl, toss together the arugula, tomatoes, pepperoncini, lemon juice, and olive oil.

3. When the quinoa is done, add it to the arugula salad, mix well, and serve.
NUTRITION: Calories: 359 Fat: 14 g. Carbs: 50 g. Protein: 10 g.

20. Coco-Nutty Brown Rice

Preparation time: 15 minutes, plus 8 hours to soak
Cooking time: 3 hours on high
Serving: 4–6
INGREDIENTS:

- 2 cups brown rice, soaked in water overnight, drained, and rinsed
- 3 cups water
- 1½ cup full-fat coconut milk
- 1 tsp. sea salt
- ½ tsp. ground ginger
- Freshly ground black pepper

DIRECTIONS:

1. In your slow cooker, combine the rice, water, coconut milk, salt, and ginger. Season with pepper and stir to incorporate the spices.
2. Cover the cooker and set to high. Cook for 3 hours and serve.

NUTRITION: Calories: 479 Fat: 19 g. Carbs: 73 g. Protein: 9 g.

21. Herbed Harvest Rice

Preparation time: 15 minutes, plus 8 hours to soak
Cooking time: 3 hours on high
Serving: 4–6
INGREDIENTS:

- 2 cups brown rice, soaked in water overnight, drained, and rinsed
- ½ small onion, chopped
- 4 cups vegetable broth
- 2 tbsp. extra-virgin olive oil
- ½ tsp. dried thyme leaves
- ½ tsp. garlic powder
- ½ cups cooked sliced mushrooms
- ½ cups dried cranberries
- ½ cup toasted pecans

DIRECTIONS:

1. In your slow cooker, combine the rice, onion, broth, olive oil, thyme, and garlic powder. Stir well. Cover the cooker and set to high. Cook for 3 hours.
2. Stir in the mushrooms, cranberries, and pecans, and serve.

NUTRITION: Calories: 546 Fat: 20 g. Carbs: 88 g. Protein: 10 g.

22. Veggie "Fried" Quinoa

Preparation time: 15 minutes or fewer
Cooking time: 4 to 6 hours on low
Serving: 4–6

INGREDIENTS:

- 2 cups quinoa, rinsed well
- 4 cups vegetable broth
- ¼ cups sliced carrots
- ¼ cups corn kernels
- ¼ cups green peas
- ¼ cups diced scallion
- 1 tbsp. sesame oil
- 1 tbsp. garlic powder
- 1 tsp. sea salt
- Dash red pepper flakes

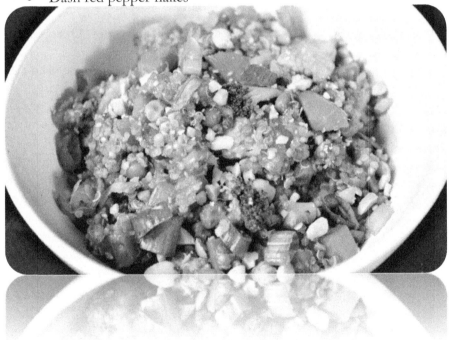

DIRECTIONS:

1. In your slow cooker, combine the quinoa, broth, carrots, corn, peas, scallion, sesame oil, garlic powder, salt, and red pepper flakes.
2. Cover the cooker and set to low. Cook for 4 to 6 hours, fluff, and serve.

NUTRITION: Calories: 387 Fat: 8 g. Carbs: 65 g. Protein: 13 g.

23. Chicken Salad Delight

Preparation time: 30 minutes
Cooking time: 5 minutes
Serving: 5

INGREDIENTS:

- 2 cups diced chicken, fat and skin removed
- 1/2 cups plain, non-fat yogurt
- 1/2 cups celery, finely chopped
- 1/4 tsp. black pepper
- 1/4 cups onion, chopped
- 1/4 cups green pepper, chopped
- 1 tsp. dried parsley
- 1 tbsp. lemon juice
- 1 tsp. dry mustard
- 3 cups water

DIRECTIONS:

1. In a pot filled with 3 cups water, boil chicken over high heat for 3–5 minutes. Drain excess water and let cool.
2. In a large mixing bowl, combine the celery, green pepper, onion, and parsley. Add chicken and toss the mixture with lemon juice.
3. In a separate bowl, mix the yogurt, black pepper, and mustard. Add the dry mixture to chicken mixture and mix thoroughly. Finally, add the lemon juice and mix again. Consume immediately.

NUTRITION: Calories: 181 Carbs: 3 g Protein: 18 g Fat: 10 g

24. Parsley Burger

Preparation time: 1 hour
Cooking time: 20 minutes
Serving: 4

INGREDIENTS:

- 1 lb. ground beef
- 1 tbsp. lemon juice
- 1/4 tsp. oregano
- 1/4 tsp. ground thyme
- 1 tbsp. parsley flakes
- 1/4 tsp. black pepper
- Vegetable oil, for greasing

DIRECTIONS:

1. In a large mixing bowl, combine the beef, lemon juice, thyme, oregano, black pepper, and parsley flakes. Mix all ingredients thoroughly.

2. Form 4 small burger patties about 3/4-inch thick each. Grease a skillet or broiler pan with vegetable oil and place the patties. Broil over medium-low heat for 15–20 minutes.

NUTRITION: Calories: 171 Carbs: 0 g. Protein: 20 g. Fat: 10 g.

25. Seasoned Pork Chops

Preparation time: 20 minutes
Cooking time: 50 minutes
Serving: 4

INGREDIENTS:
- 4 4-oz lean pork chops, skin and fat removed
- 1/4 cup all-purpose white flour
- 1 tsp. black pepper
- 1/2 tsp. thyme
- 2 tbsp. canola oil
- 1/2 tsp. sage

DIRECTIONS:
1. Preheat oven by setting the temperature to 350°F. Lightly grease a baking pan with canola oil.
2. In a medium-sized mixing bowl, combine the flour, sage, thyme, and black pepper. Mix thoroughly.
3. Dredge each pork chop in flour mixture and arrange them in greased pan. Bake in the oven for 40–50 minutes or until brown and tender. Serve.

NUTRITION: Calories: 342 Carbs: 12 g. Protein: 19 g. Fat: 23 g.

26. Taco Stuffing

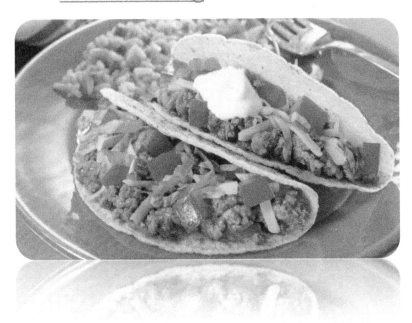

Preparation time: 30 minutes
Cooking time: 20 minutes
Serving: 8

INGREDIENTS:

- 1 1/4 lb. ground beef or turkey
- 2 tbsp. canola oil
- 1/2 tsp. ground red pepper
- 1/2 tsp. nutmeg
- 1/2 tsp. black pepper
- 1/2 tsp. Tabasco sauce
- 1 tsp. Italian seasoning
- 1 tsp. garlic powder
- 1 tsp. onion powder

To serve:

- Lettuce
- Taco shells

DIRECTIONS:

1. Heat oil over medium heat in a skillet then place ground meat and all other ingredients. Cook for 15–20 minutes or until beef is tender and everything is fully blended.
2. Stuff taco shells with 2-oz beef mixture each and top with shredded lettuce.

NUTRITION: Calories: 176 Carbs: 9 g. Protein: 14 g. Fat: 9 g.

27. Jalapeno Popper Chicken

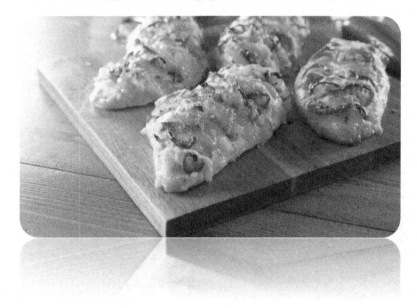

Preparation time: 5 minutes
Cooking time: 30 minutes
Serving: 8

INGREDIENTS:

- 3 tbsp. vegetable oil
- 2 tsp. fresh jalapeno peppers, seeded, finely chopped
- 2–3 lbs. chicken, cut and fat and skin removed
- 1/4 tsp. black pepper
- 1 onion, sliced into rings
- 1/2 tsp. ground nutmeg
- 1 ½ cup chicken bouillon, made from lean chicken

DIRECTIONS:

1. Heat oil in a pan over medium heat, add the chicken and cook until golden brown.
2. Add onion rings and sauté for a minute and then add the bouillon. Stir the mixture regularly and bring it to a boil.
3. Add black pepper and nutmeg. Cover the pan and simmer for 25–30 minutes or until chicken is soft and tender.
4. Stir in jalapeno peppers and simmer for another 2 minutes.

NUTRITION: Calories: 143 Carbs: 2 g. Protein: 17 g. Fat: 7 g.

28. Tuna Au Poivre

Preparation time: 30 minutes
Cooking time: 10 minutes
Serving: 4

INGREDIENTS:

- 1 tbsp. finely grated lemon zest
- 3–4 tsp. coarsely ground black pepper
- 2 garlic cloves, finely minced
- 2 tsp. dried oregano
- 1 tsp. kosher salt
- 4 6-ounce tuna
- Steaks 2 tsp.
- Olive oil 1 lemon, quartered

DIRECTIONS:

1. Place the lemon zest, black pepper, garlic, oregano, and salt on a large plate and mix to combine. Dredge both sides of the tuna in the mixture.
2. Place a large cast iron skillet over medium high heat and when it is hot, add the oil. Add the tuna and cook until browned, about 5 minutes on each side.
3. Serve immediately, garnished with the lemon quarters.

NUTRITION: Calories: 305 Fat: 11 g.Carbs: 4 g.Protein: 45 g.

29. Fish Stew

Preparation time: 30 minutes
Cooking time: 55 minutes

Serving: 8

INGREDIENTS:

- 2 tsp. olive oil
- 3 leeks, well washed, white, and light green parts only, or 1 Spanish onion, chopped
- 2 celery stalks, diced
- 2 carrots, diced peeled
- 1 fennel bulb, tough outer layers removed, trimmed, and diced
- 4 garlic cloves, finely chopped, or pressed
- 1/4 tsp. crushed red pepper
- 2 tsp. dried thyme
- 1 bay leaf
- 1/4 tsp. cayenne pepper
- 1/8 tsp. crushed saffron threads
- 1 28 ounce can whole tomatoes, chopped, including liquid
- 6 cups light fish broth or non-fat chicken broth
- 1 cup dry white wine
- Strips of zest from one orange
- 1-pound cod, cubed
- 1-pound halibut, cubed

DIRECTIONS:

1. Place a large skillet over low heat and when it is hot, add the olive oil. Add the onion, celery, carrots, and fennel and cook until the onion is golden, about 10 minutes.
2. Add garlic, herbs and spices and cook for 5 minutes. Add tomatoes, fish broth, wine and orange zest and cook for 20–25 minutes.
3. Raise the heat to high and bring the mixture to a boil. Reduce the heat to low, add the cod and halibut and cook until the fish is starting to fall apart, 10–15 minutes.
4. Transfer 2 cups of the soup to a blender and process until smooth. Return to the soup.
5. Serve immediately or cover and refrigerate up to 2 days. Serve with lemon wedges and French bread toasts or croutons.

NUTRITION: Calories: 185 Fat: 4 g. Carbs: 10 g. Protein: 27 g.

30. Grilled Salmon With Fruit And Sesame Vinaigrette

Preparation time: 15 minutes
Cooking time: 10 minutes
Serving: 4

INGREDIENTS:

- 4 6-ounce salmon steaks
- 1 tsp. Kosher salt
- 1 tsp. black pepper
- 1 tsp. olive oil
- 1 garlic clove, crushed

- 1 tsp. finely chopped fresh ginger root peeled
- ½ cup chopped red onion
- 2 tbsp. sesame seeds
- 1/4 cup lemon or lime juice
- ¼ cup orange, apple, or pineapple juice
- ¼ tsp. white sugar
- 1 tbsp. balsamic vinegar
- 1 tbsp. finely chopped fresh basil or cilantro leaves
- 2 scallion greens, finely chopped
- ¼–½ tsp. kosher salt

DIRECTIONS:

1. Prepare the grill or preheat the broiler.
2. Sprinkle the salmon with the salt and pepper. When the grill is hot, place the steaks on the grill and cook 5–6 minutes on each side. Alternatively, place under the broiler.
3. In the meantime, place a large skillet over medium heat and when it is hot, add the oil.
4. Add the garlic, ginger root, onion, and sesame seeds and cook until the vegetables are soft and the seeds are lightly browned, about 5 minutes.
5. Off heat, add the juices, sugar, vinegar, basil or cilantro, scallion greens, salt, and pepper. When the steaks are ready, top with the vinaigrette. Serve immediately.

NUTRITION: Calories: 380 Fat: 207 Fat: 23 g. Carbs: 7 g.Protein: 35 g.

31. Minty Melon with Vinegar

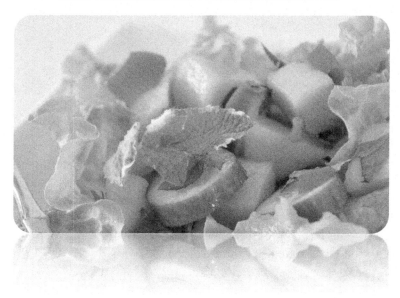

Preparation Time: 5 minutes
Cooking time: 0 minutes
Servings: 4
INGREDIENTS:
Dressing:
- 3 tablespoons olive oil
- 2 tablespoons red wine vinegar
- Sea salt, to taste

Salad:
- 1 honeydew melon, rind removed, flesh cut into 1-inch cubes
- ½ cantaloupe, rind removed, flesh cut into 1-inch cubes
- 3 stalks celery, sliced
- ½ red onion, thinly sliced
- ¼ cup chopped fresh mint

DIRECTIONS:
Make the Dressing
  1. In a small bowl, whisk the olive oil and red wine vinegar. Season with sea salt and set it aside.
Make the Salad
  2. In a large bowl, combine the honeydew, cantaloupe, celery, red onion, and mint.
  3. Add the dressing and toss to combine.
NUTRITION: Calories: 223 Fat: 11g Protein: 2g Carbs: 32g

32. Mixed Greens Salad with Honeyed Dressing

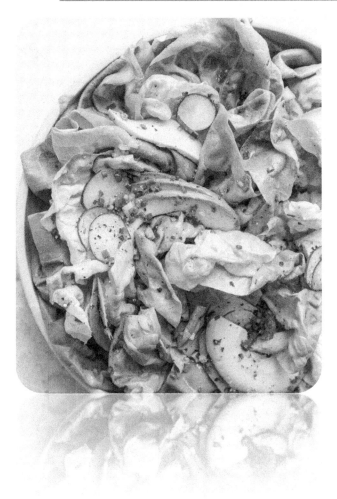

Preparation Time: 10 minutes
Cooking time: 0 minutes
Servings: 4
INGREDIENTS:
Dressing:

- ½ cup pitted Rainier cherries
- ¼ cup olive oil
- 2 tablespoons freshly squeezed lemon juice
- 2 tablespoons raw honey
- 1 teaspoon chopped fresh basil
- Pinch sea salt

Salad:

- 4 cups lightly blanched broccoli florets
- 2 cups mixed greens

- 1 cup snow peas
- ½ English cucumber, quartered lengthwise and sliced
- ½ red onion, thinly sliced

DIRECTIONS:

Make the Dressing

1. In a blender, combine the cherries, olive oil, lemon juice, honey, and basil. Pulse until smooth. Season with sea salt and set it aside.

Make the Salad

2. In a large bowl, toss the broccoli, greens, snow peas, cucumber, and red onion with the dressing to coat.

NUTRITION: Calories: 189 Fat: 13g Protein: 3g Carbs: 18g

33. <u>Apricot Salad with Mustardy Dressing</u>

Preparation Time: 10 minutes
Cooking time: 0 minutes
Servings: 4

INGREDIENTS:

Dressing:

- ¼ cup olive oil
- 2 tablespoons balsamic vinegar
- 2 teaspoons whole-grain Dijon mustard
- 1 teaspoon chopped fresh thyme
- Sea salt, to taste

Salad:

- 4 cups mixed greens
- 1 cup arugula
- ½ red onion, thinly sliced
- 16 ounces (454 g) cooked turkey breast, chopped
- 3 apricots, pitted and each fruit cut into 8 pieces
- ½ cup chopped pecans

DIRECTIONS:

Make the Dressing

1. In a small bowl, whisk the olive oil, balsamic vinegar, mustard, and thyme. Season with sea salt and set it aside.

Make the Salad

2. In a large bowl, toss together the mixed greens, arugula, and red onion with ¾ of the dressing. Arrange the dressed salad on a serving platter.

3. Top the greens with the turkey, apricots, and pecans. Drizzle with the remaining fourth of the dressing and serve.

NUTRITION: Calories: 305 Fat: 20g Protein: 21g Carbs: 12g

34. Potato Caraway with Lemony Fillet

Preparation Time: 10 minutes
Cooking time: 15 minutes
Servings: 2

INGREDIENTS:

- 1 cup peeled sweet potatoes
- 12 ounces (340 g) smoked mackerel fillets, skin removed
- 2 green onions, finely sliced
- 1 cup cooked beetroot, sliced into wedges
- 2 tablespoons finely chopped dill
- 2 tablespoons olive oil
- Juice of 1 lemon, zest of half
- 1 teaspoon crushed caraway seeds

DIRECTIONS:

1. Place the potatoes in a small saucepan of boiling water and simmer for 15 minutes over medium-high heat or until fork-tender. Cool and cut into thick slices.
2. Flake the mackerel into a bowl and add the cooled potatoes, green onions, beetroot and dill.
3. In a separate bowl, whisk together the olive oil, lemon juice, caraway seeds and black pepper.
4. Pour over the salad and toss well to coat. Scatter over the lemon zest. Pack into plastic containers and chill for later, or enjoy straight away.

NUTRITION: Calories: 530 Fat: 38g Protein: 34g Carbs: 13g

35. Vinegary Berry with Orange Salad

Preparation Time: 10 minutes
Cooking time: 0 minutes
Servings: 1

INGREDIENTS:

- 1 cup fresh spinach, leaves trimmed and coarsely chopped
- 1 orange, peeled and sliced
- 1 cup chopped fresh cranberries
- 2 tablespoons red wine vinegar
- 4 teaspoons olive oil
- 2 teaspoons peeled and grated ginger
- 1 pinch of black pepper

DIRECTIONS:

1. Grab a salad bowl and mix the vinegar and olive oil until blended and then add in the cranberries and ginger, adding pepper to taste.
2. Add the spinach and orange slices to the dressing and then toss to coat. Chill before serving.

NUTRITION: Calories: 298 Fat: 18g Protein: 2g Carbs: 32g

36. Cucumber and Spinach with Chicken Salad

Preparation Time: 10 minutes
Cooking time: 15 minutes
Servings: 2
INGREDIENTS:
- 1 tablespoon extra-virgin olive oil
- 2 skinless chicken breasts, chopped
- 2 carrots, sliced
- ½ large onion, chopped
- 2 teaspoons cumin seeds
- ½ avocado, chopped
- 1 lime, juiced
- ½ cucumber, chopped
- ½ cup fresh spinach
- 1 mason jar

DIRECTIONS:
1. In a skillet, heat the oil over medium heat and then cook the chicken for 10 to 15 minutes until browned and cooked through. Remove and place to one side to cool.
2. Add the carrots and onion and continue to cook for 5 to 10 minutes or until soft.
3. Add the cumin seeds in a separate pan over high heat and toast until they're brown before crushing them in a pestle and mortar or blender.
4. Put them into the pan with the veggies and turn off the heat. Add the avocado and lime juice into a food processor and blend until creamy.
5. Layer the jar with half of the avocado and lime mixture, then the cumin roasted veggies, and then the chicken, packing it all in.
6. Top with the tomatoes, cucumbers, and the cilantro and spinach, refrigerating for 20 minutes before serving.

NUTRITION: Calories: 522 Fat: 22g Protein: 64g Carbs: 17g

37. Lemony Zucchini with Vinegary Salmon

Preparation Time: 10 minutes
Cooking time: 14 minutes
Servings: 2
INGREDIENTS:
- 2 skinless salmon fillets
- 2 cups seasonal greens
- ½ cup sliced zucchini
- 1 tablespoon balsamic vinegar
- 2 tablespoons extra-virgin olive oil
- 2 sprigs thyme, torn from the stem

- 1 lemon, juiced

DIRECTIONS:

1. Preheat the broiler to medium-high heat. Broil the salmon in parchment paper with some oil, lemon and pepper for 10 minutes.
2. Slice the zucchini and sauté for 4 to 5 minutes with the oil in a pan over medium heat.
3. Build the salad by creating a bed of zucchini and topping with flaked salmon. Drizzle with balsamic vinegar and sprinkle with thyme.

NUTRITION: Calories: 531 Fat: 27g Protein: 67g Carbs: 5g

38. Carrot Salad with Lemony Cashew Dressing

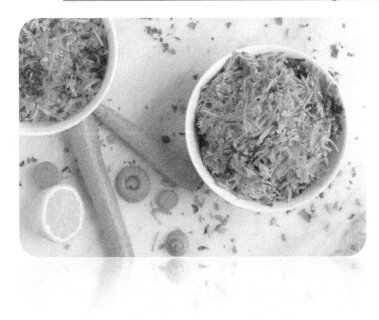

Preparation Time: 5 minutes
Cooking time: 0 minutes
Servings: 6

INGREDIENTS:

Salad:

- 2 carrots, grated
- 1 large head green or red cabbage, sliced thin

Dressing:

- 1 cup cashews, soaked in water for at least 4 hours, drained
- ¼ cup freshly squeezed lemon juice
- ¾ teaspoon sea salt
- ½ cup water

DIRECTIONS:

1. Combine the carrots and cabbage in a large serving bowl. Toss to combine well.
2. Put the ingredients for the dressing in a food processor, then pulse until creamy and smooth.

3. Dress the salad, then refrigerate for at least 1 hour before serving.
NUTRITION: Calories: 208 Fat: 11g Protein: 7g Carbs: 25g

39. Milky Carrot with Oniony Ginger Soup

Preparation Time: 5 minutes
Cooking time: 28 minutes
Servings: 6-8
INGREDIENTS:
- 4½ cups plus 2 tablespoons water, divided
- 1 large onion, peeled and roughly chopped
- 8 carrots, peeled and roughly chopped
- 1½-inch piece fresh ginger, sliced thin
- 1¼ teaspoons sea salt
- 2 cups unsweetened coconut milk

DIRECTIONS:
1. Add 2 tablespoons of water to a large pot, then add the onion and sauté over medium heat for 4 minutes or until translucent.
2. Add the carrots, ginger, salt, and remaining water to the pot. Bring to a boil, then reduce the heat to low. Cover and simmer for 20 minutes.
3. When the simmering is over, open the lid, then mix in the coconut milk and cook for 4 more minutes.
4. Pour the soup in a blender, then pulse to purée until creamy and smooth. Serve the soup in a large bowl immediately.

NUTRITION: Calories: 228 Fat: 19g Protein: 3g Carbs: 15g

40. Garlicky Broccoli with Cashew Soup

Preparation Time: 10 minutes
Cooking time: 25 minutes
Servings: 6
INGREDIENTS:
- 5 cups plus 2 tablespoons water, divided
- 1 onion, finely chopped
- 4 garlic cloves, finely chopped
- 4 broccoli heads with stalks, heads cut into florets and stalks roughly chopped
- 1½ teaspoons sea salt, plus additional as needed
- 1 cup cashews, soaked in water for at least 4 hours, drained

DIRECTIONS:
1. Add 2 tablespoons of water to a large pot, then add the onion and garlic and sauté over medium heat for 5 minutes or until the onion is translucent.
2. Add the broccoli, salt, and remaining water. Bring to a boil, then reduce the heat to low. Cover and simmer for 20 minutes.

3. Pour the soup in a blender, then add the cashews. Pulse to purée until creamy and smooth. Pour the soup in a large bowl and serve immediately.

NUTRITION: Calories: 224 Fat: 11g Protein: 11g Carbs: 26g

41. Squashy Carrot and Celery Soup

Preparation Time: 5 minutes
Cooking time: 30 minutes
Servings: 6

INGREDIENTS:
- 4½ cups plus 2 tablespoons water, divided
- 1 onion, roughly chopped
- 1 large butternut squash, washed, peeled, ends trimmed, halved, seeded, and cut into ½-inch chunks
- 3 carrots, peeled and roughly chopped
- 2 celery stalks, roughly chopped
- 1 teaspoon sea salt, or to taste

DIRECTIONS:
1. Add 2 tablespoons of water to a large pot, then add the onion and sauté over medium heat for 5 minutes or until tender.
2. Add the butternut squash, carrots, celery, salt, and remaining water. Bring to a boil. Reduce the heat to low, then simmer for 25 minutes or until the squash is soft.
3. Pour the soup in a food processor, then pulse to purée until creamy and smooth. Pour the soup in a large bowl and serve immediately.

NUTRITION: Calories: 104 Fat: 0g Protein: 2g Carbs: 27g

42. Mixed Greens Soup with Coconut Milk

Preparation Time: 10 minutes
Cooking time: 15 minutes
Servings: 4-6

INGREDIENTS:
- 2 cups unsweetened coconut milk
- 3 cups water
- 1½ teaspoons sea salt, or to taste
- 1 bunch fresh parsley, rinsed, stemmed and roughly chopped
- 4 cups tightly packed kale, rinsed, stemmed, and roughly chopped
- 4 cups tightly packed spinach, rinsed, stemmed and roughly chopped
- 4 cups tightly packed collard greens, rinsed, stemmed and roughly chopped

DIRECTIONS:
1. Pour the coconut milk and water in a large pot, then sprinkle with salt. Bring to a boil over high heat. Reduce the heat to low.

2. Add 1 cup of each greens to the pot and cook for 5 minutes or until wilted. Repeat with the remaining greens. When all the greens are wilted, simmer for 10 minutes.
3. Pour the soup in a blender, then pulse until creamy and smooth. Pour the soup in a large bowl and serve immediately.

NUTRITION: Calories: 334 Fat: 29g Protein: 7g Carbs: 18g

43. Onion Chipotle Soup with Sage

Preparation Time: 10 minutes
Cooking time: 11 minutes
Servings: 4

INGREDIENTS:
- 2 tablespoons extra-virgin olive oil
- 1 onion, chopped
- 2 garlic cloves, cut into 1/8-inch-thick slices
- 1 (15-ounce / 425-g) can pumpkin purée
- 4 cups low-sodium vegetable broth
- 2 teaspoons chipotle powder
- 1 teaspoon sea salt
- ½ teaspoon freshly ground black pepper
- 2 tablespoons coconut oil
- 12 sage leaves, stemmed

DIRECTIONS:
1. Heat the olive oil in a large pot over high heat until shimmering. Add the onion and garlic and sauté for 5 minutes or until the onion browns.
2. Pour in the pumpkin purée and vegetable broth, then sprinkle with chipotle powder, salt, and ground black pepper. Stir to mix well.
3. Bring to a boil. Reduce the heat to low and simmer for 5 minutes. Meanwhile, heat the coconut oil in a nonstick skillet over high heat.
4. Add the sage leaves to the skillet and cook for 1 minute or until crispy.
5. When the simmering is complete, divide the soup in four serving bowls, then garnish each bowl with 3 crispy sage leaves and serve.

NUTRITION: Calories: 380 Fat: 20g Protein: 10g Carbs: 45g

44. Pears with Peppered Fennel Soup

Preparation Time: 10 minutes
Cooking time: 13 minutes
Servings: 4-6

INGREDIENTS:
- 2 tablespoons extra-virgin olive oil
- 1 fennel bulb, cut into ¼-inch-thick slices
- 2 leeks, white part only, sliced

- 2 pears, peeled, cored, and cut into ½-inch cubes
- 1 teaspoon sea salt
- ¼ teaspoon freshly ground black pepper
- ½ cup cashews
- 3 cups low-sodium vegetable broth
- 2 cups packed spinach

DIRECTIONS:
1. Heat the olive oil in a large pot over high heat until shimmering. Add the fennel and leeks and sauté for 5 minutes or until tender.
2. Add the pears and sprinkle with salt and pepper. Sauté for another 3 minutes.
3. Add the cashews and vegetable broth. Bring to a boil. Reduce the heat to low. Cover and simmer for 5 minutes.
4. Pour the soup in a blender and add the spinach. Pulse until creamy and smooth. Pour the soup in a large serving bowl and serve immediately.

NUTRITION: Calories: 266 Fat: 15g Protein: 5g Carbs: 33g

45. Scallion with Minty Cucumber Salad

Preparation Time: 15 minutes
Cooking time: 0 minutes
Servings: 4

INGREDIENTS:
- 1 bunch radishes, sliced thin
- 1 English cucumber, peeled and diced
- 2 cups packed spinach
- 3 large tomatoes, diced
- 1 tablespoon chopped fresh mint
- 1 tablespoon chopped fresh parsley
- 2 scallions, sliced
- 2 garlic cloves, minced
- 1 cup unsweetened plain almond yogurt
- 1 tablespoon apple cider vinegar
- 3 tablespoons freshly squeezed lemon juice
- 1 tablespoon sumac
- 2 tablespoons extra-virgin olive oil
- 1 teaspoon sea salt
- ¼ teaspoon freshly ground black pepper

DIRECTIONS:
1. Combine all the ingredients in a large salad bowl. Toss to mix well, then serve immediately.

NUTRITION: Calories: 195 Fat: 14g Protein: 4g Carbs: 15g

46. Beef & Sweet Potato Enchilada Casserole

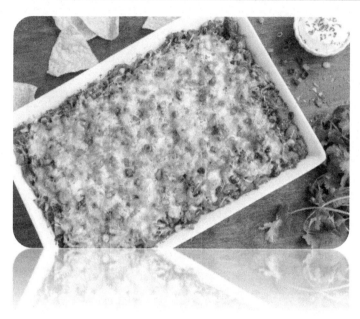

Preparation Time: 20 minutes
Cooking time: 20 minutes
Servings: 10
INGREDIENTS:

- 2 sweet potatoes
- 1 pound ground beef
- 1 can black beans, drained
- 1 cup frozen corn
- 1 can red enchilada sauce
- 4 tablespoon chopped fresh cilantro
- 2 teaspoon ground cumin
- 1 teaspoon garlic powder
- 1 teaspoon onion powder
- 12 corn tortillas
- 1 small can diced olives
- 4 tablespoons coconut cream

DIRECTIONS:

1. Peel and cook the sweet potatoes; mash and mix with 2 tablespoons of cilantro. Cook the ground beef and then stir in beans, corn, sauce and spices until well combined.

2. Layer half of the meat mixture in a 9x13-inch pan and top with half of corn tortilla; sprinkle with half of the coconut cream and repeat the layers.
3. Top with sweet potatoes, olives and cilantro. Cover with the remaining cream and bake at 350°F for about 25 minutes or until cheese is melted.

NUTRITION: Calories: 315 Fat: 8.2 g Carbs: 5.4 g Protein: 31.6 g

47. Delicious Buckwheat with Mushrooms & Green Onions

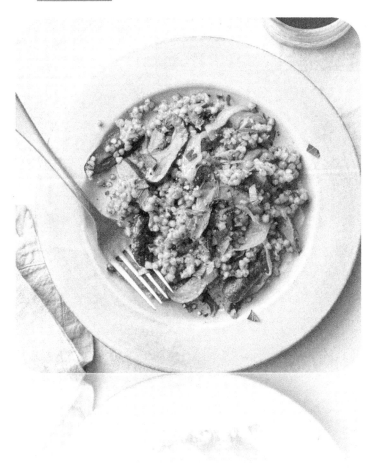

Preparation Time: 20 minutes
Cooking time: 35 minutes
Servings: 6

INGREDIENTS:

- 1 cup uncooked buckwheat
- 2 cup water
- 2 cups mushrooms
- 1 red onion, chopped
- 1 cup chopped green onions

- 3 tablespoons butter
- A pinch of salt and pepper

DIRECTIONS:
1. Combine buckwheat, salt, and water in a pan   bring to a boil; cook for 25 minutes or until liquid is absorbed.
2. Melt butter in a pan and fry in red onion until tender; stir in mushrooms and cook for about 5 minutes or until golden brown.
3. Stir in cooked buckwheat and remove from heat. Serve topped with freshly chopped green onions.

NUTRITION: Calories: 166 Fat: 6.8 g Carbs: 20.1 g Protein: 5.1 g

48. Yummy Chicken and Sweet Potato Stew

Preparation Time: 15 minutes
Cooking time: 4-8 hours
Servings: 4-6

INGREDIENTS:
- 1-pound boneless chicken breasts, with skin removed and cut into chunks
- 1 Vidalia onion, chopped
- 4 cloves garlic, crushed
- 3 carrots, peeled and diced
- 1 sweet potato, peeled and cut into cubes
- 2 cups chicken broth, preferably homemade
- 3 tablespoons balsamic vinegar
- 2-4 tablespoons tomato paste
- 2 teaspoons whole grain mustard
- 2 cups fresh baby spinach
- Freshly ground pepper and salt to taste

DIRECTIONS:
1. Combine all the ingredients in your slow cooker and stir well until evenly combined. Cover and cook on low for 6 to 8 hours or on high for 4-5 hours.
2. When left with a few minutes of cook time, stir in the baby spinach. Serve hot.

NUTRITION: Calories: 139 Fat: 3.7g Carbs: 2.6 g Protein: 5.4 g

49. Healthy Fried Brown Rice with Peas & Prawns

Preparation Time: 10 minutes
Cooking time: 10 minutes
Servings: 8

INGREDIENTS:
- 1/2 cup frozen pea
- 2 cups cooked brown rice

- 2 teaspoons extra-virgin olive oil
- 1 red chilli, sliced
- 2 garlic cloves, sliced
- 1 red onion, sliced
- 1 cup large peeled prawn
- 1 bunch coriander, chopped
- 1 tablespoon fish sauce
- 1 tablespoon dark soy sauce
- 4 large eggs
- 1 tablespoon chilli sauce

DIRECTIONS:

1. Sauté garlic, onion and chilli in hot oil in a skillet for about 3 minutes or until golden; stir in prawns for about 1 minute and then toss in peas and rice.
2. Cook until heated through. Stir in fish sauce, soy sauce and coriander and cook for a minute. Remove from heat and keep warm. Heat oil in a pan and fry the eggs; season.
3. Divide rice mixture among four serving plates and top each with a fried egg. Serve with chili sauce topped with coriander.

NUTRITION: Calories: 278 Fat: 4.3 g Carbs: 44.9 g Protein: 8.3 g

50. Asparagus Quinoa & Steak Bowl

Preparation Time: 10 minutes
Cooking time: 15 minutes
Servings: 4

INGREDIENTS:

- 1-1/2 cups white quinoa
- Olive oil cooking spray
- 3/4-pound lean steak, diced
- 1/2 tsp. low-sodium steak seasoning
- 1/2 cup chopped red bell pepper
- 1/2 cup chopped red onion
- 1 cup frozen asparagus cuts
- 2 ½ tbsp. soy sauce

DIRECTIONS:

1. Follow package instructions to cook quinoa. In the meantime, coat a large skillet with cooking spray and heat over medium high heat.
2. Sprinkle beef with the steak seasoning and cook in the skillet for about 3 minutes; add bell pepper and red onion and cook for 3 minutes more or until beef is browned.
3. Add asparagus and continue cooking for 4 minutes or until asparagus is heated through. Stir soy sauce to the quinoa until well combined and toss it with the beef mixture before serving.

NUTRITION: Calories: 325 Fat: 8.2 g Carbs: 17.4 g Protein: 26.3 g

51. Seared Lemon Steak with Vegetables Stir-Fry

Preparation Time: 15 minutes
Cooking time: 10 minutes
Servings: 3-4
INGREDIENTS:

- 1-pound lean steak
- ¼ cup fresh lemon juice
- 1 tablespoon lemon zest
- 1 ½ cups almond milk
- 2 teaspoons coconut oil
- 1 cup chopped red onion
- 4 cloves garlic, minced
- 2 cups shiitake mushrooms, diced
- 3 medium zucchinis
- 1 green pepper bell
- 1 red pepper bell
- 3 tomatoes
- 1 teaspoon curry powder
- 1 tablespoon ginger
- ¼ teaspoon salt
- ¼ teaspoon pepper

DIRECTIONS:
1. Rub the meat with lemon juice and sprinkle salt, lemon zest, and cayenne pepper; heat half of coconut oil in a skillet set over medium heat and sear in the meat for about 6 minutes per side or until cooked through and golden browned on the outside.
2. Keep the meat warm wrapped in a foil. Dice zucchinis, bell peppers, tomatoes, and beans in bite-size pieces.
3. Heat oil in a pan and fry the red onion and garlic; add in mushrooms, zucchini, and bell peppers; fry for 3 minutes more.
4. Stir in almond milk and tomatoes and cook for a few minutes. Season with ginger, curry powder, salt and pepper. Serve topped with sliced steak.

NUTRITION: Calories: 406 Fat: 33.6 g Carbs: 20.2 g Protein: 15.1 g

52. Vegetable Tabbouleh

Preparation Time: 5 minutes
Cooking time: 10 minutes
Servings: 2
INGREDIENTS:

- 1 cup broccoli florets
- 1 chopped carrots

- 1 cup shredded cabbage
- 1 teaspoon sesame seeds
- A pinch of salt and pepper
- 1 cup cooked quinoa
- 1 cucumber, sliced
- ¼ cup fresh lemon juice
- Handful cilantro

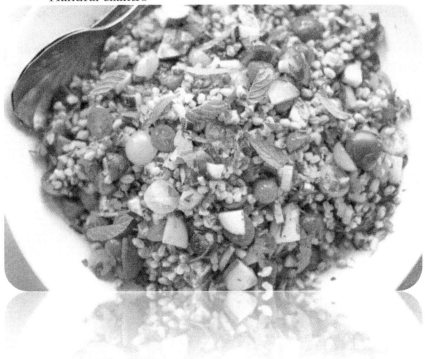

DIRECTIONS:
1. Heat oil in a skillet set over medium heat until hot, but not smoky; stir-fry in red onions, garlic, broccoli florets, chopped fresh chili, chopped carrots, shredded cabbage, and sesame seeds.
2. Cook for about 5 minutes or until the veggies are crisp tender. Season with salt and pepper and remove from heat.
3. Serve with cooked quinoa topped with cucumber and chopped cilantro; drizzle with fresh lemon juice for a healthy flavorful meal.

NUTRITION: Calories: 447 Carbs: 48g Fat: 27g Protein: 9g

53. <u>Peppered Steak with Cherry Tomatoes</u>

Preparation Time: 10 minutes
Cooking time: 10 minutes
Servings: 4
INGREDIENTS:

- 4 (250g) lean beef steaks

- 1 tablespoon extra-virgin olive oil
- 2 tablespoons pepper
- 1 bunch rocket
- 2 cups cherry tomatoes
- 4 cups green salad
- olive oil cooking spray

DIRECTIONS:
1. Brush the steak with oil. Place the pepper on a large plate and press the steaks into the pepper until well coated.
2. Pre heat your chargrill or barbecue grill on medium high and barbecue the steaks for about 5 minutes per side or until cooked well. Transfer the cooed steaks to a plate and keep warm.
3. In the meantime, sprat the tomatoes with oil and barbecue them, turning occasionally, for about 5 minutes or until tender.
4. Arrange the rocket on serving plates and add steaks and tomatoes; serve with green salad.

NUTRITION: Calories: 237 Fat: 11.1g Carbs: 10.7g Protein: 14.8g

54. Grilled Chicken Breast with Non-Fat Yogurt

Preparation Time: 2 hours
Cooking time: 10 minutes
Servings: 3
INGREDIENTS:
For the Grilled Chicken:
- 3 boneless chicken breast halves, skinned
- 1 clove garlic, minced
- 1 tablespoon lemon juice, freshly squeezed
- 1 teaspoon extra virgin olive oil
- 1 teaspoon dried oregano
- Salt and freshly ground black pepper, to taste

For the yogurt:
- 1 cup nonfat Greek yogurt
- 1 clove garlic, minced
- 1 tsp. fresh dill, minced
- ½ cup cucumber, very thinly sliced or shredded

DIRECTIONS:
1. Use a sharp knife to gently slice through the thickest part of the chicken breast with cutting all the way through so you are able to open it up like a book. Do this for the other two halves.
2. Marinate the chicken with the remaining chicken ingredients in a large bowl. Cover with cling wrap and set in the fridge for 1 ½ to 2 hours. Preheat your grill to medium-high heat.
3. Take out the chicken from the marinade. Lightly grease your grill rack then place the breasts on top.
4. Cook for about 3 minutes on each side or until done to desire. Meanwhile, combine all the yogurt ingredients in a medium bowl.

5. To serve, serve each breast on a large plate. Place a dollop of the nutty yogurt on the side. Enjoy!

NUTRITION: Calories: 318 Fat: 33. G Carbs: 8 g Protein: 37.2g

55. Delicious Low Fat Chicken Curry

Preparation Time: 10 minutes
Cooking time: 20 minutes
Servings: 1

INGREDIENTS:

- 100 grams chicken, diced
- ¼ cup chicken broth
- Pinch of turmeric
- Dash of onion powder
- 1 tablespoon minced red onion
- Pinch of garlic powder
- ¼ teaspoon curry powder
- Pinch of sea salt
- Pinch of pepper
- Stevia, optional
- Pinch of cayenne

DIRECTIONS:

1. In a small saucepan, stir spices in chicken broth until dissolved; stir in chicken, garlic, onion, and stevia and cook until chicken is cooked through and liquid is reduced by half. Serve hot.

NUTRITION: Calories: 170 Fat: 3.5 g Carbs: 2.3 g Protein: 30.5 g

56. Tilapia with Mushroom Sauce

Preparation Time: 15 minutes
Cooking time: 25 minutes
Servings: 4

INGREDIENTS:

- 4 ounces tilapia fillets
- 2 teaspoon arrow root
- 1 cup mushrooms, sliced
- 1 clove garlic, finely chopped
- 1 small onion, thinly sliced
- 1 teaspoon extra-virgin olive oil
- ½ cup fresh parsley, roughly chopped
- 1 teaspoon thyme leaves, finely chopped
- ½ cup water
- A pinch of freshly ground black pepper

- A pinch of sea salt

DIRECTIONS:
1. Preheat your oven to 350°F. Add extra virgin olive oil to a frying pan set over medium heat; sauté onion, garlic and mushrooms for about 4 minutes or until mushrooms are slightly tender.
2. Stir in arrowroot, sea salt, thyme and pepper and cook for about 1 minute. Stir in water until thickened; stir in parsley and cook for 1 minute more.
3. Place the fillets on a baking tray lined with parchment paper; cover the fish with mushroom sauce and bake for about 20 minutes or until the fish is cooked through.

NUTRITION: Calories: 177 Fat: 3.7 g Carbs: 3.3 g Protein: 14.9 g

57. Ginger Chicken with Veggies

Preparation Time: 10 minutes
Cooking time: 5 minutes
Servings: 4

INGREDIENTS:
- 2 cup skinless, boneless, and cooked chicken breast meat, diced
- 1 teaspoon extra virgin olive
- 1 teaspoon powdered ginger
- 2 red onions, sliced
- 4 cloves garlic, minced
- 1 bell pepper, sliced
- 1 cup thinly sliced carrots
- 1 cup finely chopped celery
- 1 cup chicken broth (not salted)

DIRECTIONS:
1. Add the oil to a skillet set over medium heat; sauté onion and garlic until translucent. Stir in the remaining ingredients and simmer for a few minutes or until the veggies are tender.

NUTRITION: Calories: 425 Fat: 21.1g Carbs: 6.5 g Protein: 52g

58. Hot Lemon Prawns

Preparation Time: 15 minutes
Cooking time: 12 minutes
Servings: 4

INGREDIENTS:
- 400g raw king prawns
- 1 teaspoon coconut oil
- 40g ginger, grated
- 2-4 green chillies, halved
- 4 curry leaves

- 1 onion, sliced
- 4 teaspoons lemon juice
- 3-4 teaspoons red chilli powder
- 2 teaspoons turmeric
- 1 teaspoon black pepper
- 40g grated coconut
- ½ small bunch coriander

DIRECTIONS:
1. Rinse the prawns and pat dry with a kitchen towel; add them to a large bowl and then toss in chili powder, turmeric, grated ginger, and lemon juice; set aside.
2. Heat oil in a saucepan and sauté onion, ginger, chilli, and curry leaves for about 10 minutes or until translucent. Stir in black pepper and then add in prawns along with the marinade.
3. Cook for about 2 minutes or until cooked through. Season and drizzle with extra lemon juice. Serve the prawns sprinkled with coriander and grated coconut. Enjoy!

NUTRITION: Calories: 171 Fat: 8 g Carbs: 4 g Protein: 19 g

59. Delicious Chicken Tikka Skewers

Preparation Time: 20 minutes
Cooking time: 20 minutes
Servings: 4

INGREDIENTS:
- 4 boneless, skinless chicken breasts, diced
- 2 tablespoons hot curry paste
- 1 red onion, sliced
- ½ cucumber, sliced
- For the cucumber salad
- 250g pack cherry tomatoes
- 50g pack lamb's lettuce
- juice 1 lemon
- 150g nonfat Greek yogurt
- handful chopped coriander leaves

DIRECTIONS:
1. Soak skewers in a bowl of water.
2. In a bowl, mix together curry paste and yogurt; add in chicken and then marinate for 1 hour.
3. Meanwhile, toss together red onion, cucumber, coriander, and fresh lemon juice in a bowl. Refrigerate until ready to serve.
4. Thread chicken and cherry tomatoes on the skewers and grill for about 20 minutes or until cooked through and golden browned on the outside.
5. Add the lettuce into the salad and stir in mix well; divide among serving bowls and top each with two chicken skewers. Enjoy!

NUTRITION: Calories: 234 Fat: 4 g Carbs: 9.7 g Protein: 40 g

60. Grilled Chicken with Salad Wrap

Preparation Time: 5 minutes
Cooking time: 0 minutes
Servings: 2

INGREDIENTS:

- 2 lettuce leaves
- ½ coddled egg
- 1 cup diced cherry tomatoes
- 6 cups chopped curly kale
- 8 ounces sliced grilled chicken
- 1 clove garlic, minced
- 1/2 teaspoon Dijon mustard
- 1 teaspoon raw honey
- 1 teaspoon olive oil
- 1/8 cup fresh lemon juice
- Salt & pepper

DIRECTIONS:

1. In a large bowl, whisk together half of the egg, honey, mustard, minced garlic, olive oil, fresh lemon juice, salt and pepper until well combined.
2. Add in cherry tomatoes, chicken and kale and toss to coat well; spread the mixture onto lettuce leaves and roll to form wraps. Slice in half and serve right away!

NUTRITION: Calories: 386 Fat: 2.6 g Carbs: 28.5 g Protein: 32.5 g

61. Pork Egg Roll Soup

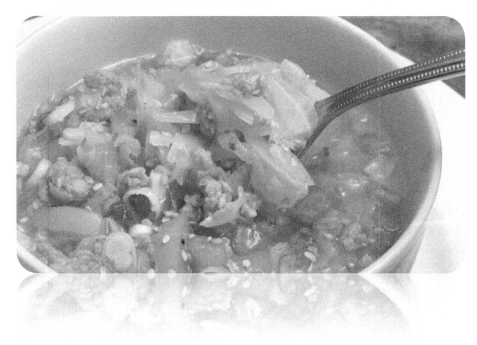

Preparation Time: 10 minutes
Cooking time: 2 hours
Servings: 4

INGREDIENTS:

- Avocado oil (1 tbsp.)
- Ribbed pork (1 lb.)
- 2 medium onion (chopped)
- Meat broth (5 ½ cups)
- Cabbage (1 ½ lb., chopped)
- Carrot (1lb. shredded)
- Garlic (1 clove, chopped)
- Salt (1 tsp.)
- ginger (1 1/2 tsp, ground)
- Coconut sauce (3/4 cup)
- Cornstarch (3 tbsp.)

DIRECTIONS:

1. Set your stock pot over medium heat, add your oil and allow to get hot. Once hot, add in your meat then brown on all sides.

2. Add your onions, cabbage, broth, garlic, salt, ginger, and coconut sauce. Cook on low heat for 1 hour and 30 minutes.
3. Combine 3 tbsp. of cornstarch to 2/3 cup of broth together in a small bowl, add to soup, and return to cook (at a low temperature) for another 30 minutes. Serve.

NUTRITION: Calories 218 Fat 12.9g Protein 18.7g Carbs 7.6g

62. Pork Casserole

Preparation Time: 15 minutes
Cooking time: 1 hour & 40 minutes
Servings: 4

INGREDIENTS:
- 2 tbsp olive oil
- 1 lb pork, cut into cubes
- 3 onions, quarter cut
- 1 yellow pepper, cut into thick strips
- 4 red peppers, quarter cut
- 1 lb ripe tomatoes, quarter cut
- 5 tbsp sun-dried tomato paste
- 6 oz green olives
- 1 can (2 oz) black olives
- 2 ½ cups water
- 1 cup red wine
- 6 tbsp fresh oregano, chopped

DIRECTIONS:
1. Set a pot on medium heat. Pour the olive oil into the pot. Brown the pork for 5 minutes.
2. Add the onions, yellow peppers, and red peppers. Sauté for 3 minutes. Add the rest of the ingredients, except the fresh oregano.
3. Cover the pot. Cook for an 1hour and 40 minutes. Garnish with fresh oregano before serving.

NUTRITION: Calories 400 Fat 10.5g Protein 28.5g Carbs 22.5g

63. Delicious Pork Roast Baracoa

Preparation Time: 10 minutes
Cooking time: 8 hours
Servings:

INGREDIENTS:
- 7 pounds of pork roast, cut into chunks
- 1 can diced green chilies
- 6 cloves minced garlic
- 1 tbsp cumin
- 8 tsp salt

- Juice from 3 different limes
- 1 diced onion
- 2-3 chopped chipotles in adobo sauce
- 9 tbsp apple cider vinegar
- 1 tbsp coriander
- 1 tsp black pepper
- ½ cup of fat free pork broth of choice

DIRECTIONS:
1. Take all of your ingredients and put them into the slow cooker, mixing them. Cook on low for 6-8 hours or until your meat can be shredded.
2. Shred the meat and mix with the juices. Serve with a fork for best results.

NUTRITION: Calories 283 Fat 11.7g Protein 37.1g Carbs 8g

64. Swedish Meatballs & Mushrooms Gravy

Preparation Time: 15 minutes
Cooking time: 40 minutes
Servings: 6-8

INGREDIENTS:
- 1 onion (large), chopped
- 1 pound/ 450 grams ground pork
- 1 pound/450 grams ground pork
- 1 teaspoon sage (dried)
- ½ cup coconut milk, bone broth, or water
- ½ teaspoon mace (ground)
- ½ teaspoon sea salt
- ¼ cup parsley (fresh), minced, divided
- 10 cups (cremini/button) mushrooms, sliced
- 11 tablespoons onion (dried), chopped
- 12 tablespoons coconut aminos

DIRECTIONS:
1. In a bowl, mix the pork, pork, salt, mace, dried onion, and 3 tablespoons parsley. Form the mixture into 1-inch meatballs.
2. Put the mushrooms, fresh onion, coconut milk/broth/water, and coconut aminos in your IP. Add the meatballs.
3. Lock the lid and close the pressure valve. Set to MEAT/STEW for 35 minutes. When the timer beeps, QPR and open the lid.
4. Gently transfer the meatballs with a slotted spoon to a serving dish. Using a stick blender or a high-powered blender, puree the remaining contents of the pot.
5. Adding coconut milk/broth/water as needed to thin. Pour the gravy over the meatballs; garnish with the remaining parsley.

NUTRITION: Calories 278 Fat 12.2g Protein 37g Carbs 4g

65. Cherry & Apple Pork

Preparation Time: 10 minutes
Cooking time: 35 minutes
Servings: 4

INGREDIENTS:

- olive oil, 1 tbsp., extra virgin, plus some for squash
- 13 cups dice apple
- 2/3 cup pit cherry
- 1/3 cup diced onion
- 1/3 cup diced celery
- ½ cup apple juice, sugar free
- 1/8 teaspoon salt
- 1/8 teaspoon black pepper
- 1 1/3 pounds boneless pork loin

DIRECTIONS:

1. Combine all the ingredients in an Instant Pot and close the lid. Select the Meat/Stew function and cook for 40 minutes.
2. Do a quick release of pressure. Serve.

NUTRITION: Calories 237 Fat 12g Protein 0.7g Carbs 6g

66. Paleo Italian Pork

Preparation Time: 5 minutes
Cooking time: 2 hours & 45 minutes
Servings: 4

INGREDIENTS:

- 16 lbs. grass-fed pork roast, cut into pieces
- 1 tablespoons garlic powder
- 1 tsp onion powder
- 1 teaspoon ginger powder
- 1 teaspoon oregano
- 1 teaspoon basil
- 1 teaspoons salt
- 2 ½ cups chicken broth
- 14 tablespoons apple cider vinegar

DIRECTIONS:

1. In a bowl add garlic powder, onion powder, ginger powder, oregano, basil, and salt. Stir to fully incorporate.
2. Rub this mixture on your roast and set aside. Set a deep pot on medium heat. Once hot add your roast and allow to brown on all sides evenly (about 2 minutes per side).

3. Drizzle pork broth and apple cider vinegar into the pot. Cover with lid, set to cook on low heat for 2 hours 45 minutes. Remove pork roast from pot. Add your meat into a shallow platter.
4. Pull the meat apart using two forks. To do this use the first fork to hold the meat steady by stabbing it directing in the center of the meat.
5. Next, place the second fork into the meat where the first fork is, with the teeth facing you, then pull it towards you.
6. Repeat this process until you have shredded all the pork. Serve, and enjoy.

NUTRITION: Calories 288 Fat 11g Protein 42g Carbs 1.6g

67. Corned Pork

Preparation Time: 5 minutes
Cooking time: 2 hours & 30 minutes
Servings: 6

INGREDIENTS:
- 3-pounds corned pork brisket
- 2 cups red potatoes, whole
- 2 onions, halved
- 9-10 garlic cloves
- 2½ cups of pork broth
- 1 cabbage, chopped
- 1 bay leaf
- 2 cloves
- 12-15 peppercorns
- 2 tablespoons coriander seeds
- ¼ teaspoon cumin seeds
- 2 cinnamon sticks
- 2 tablespoons cornstarch

DIRECTIONS:
1. Transfer pork to a deep pot with onion, red potatoes, pork broth, all spices, and garlic. Covered.
2. Cook over a medium flame for 2 hours and 20 minutes. When done, add cabbage into the pot and cook on high flame for few minutes or until the cabbage is cooked.
3. After that remove pork and vegetables from your pot, leaving drippings.
4. Mix cornstarch with drippings until combined. Now whisk this mixture into the pork juices and cook it on medium flame till boiled. Reduce flame and cook for 3-4 minutes more. Serve and enjoy.

NUTRITION: Calories 379.2 Fat 10.6g Protein 59.1g Carbs 9.7g

68. Chipotle Pork Carnitas

Preparation Time: 15 minutes

Cooking time: 2 hours & 45 minutes

Servings: 8

INGREDIENTS:

- pork shoulder, blade roast, 2 lb, boneless and trimmed
- ½ tsp garlic powder
- dry adobo seasoning, ¼ tsp
- 2 bay leaves
- 3 chipotle peppers
- 1 ¾ cup chicken stock
- Oregano, ¼ tsp, dried
- 4 tsp salt
- ½ tsp sazon
- 1 tsp cumin
- 5 garlic cloves, cut into slivers
- Black pepper to taste

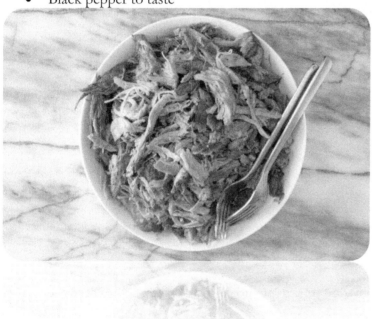

DIRECTIONS:

1. In a large pan, brown the pork on all sides over the high heat for 5 minutes. Remove pork from pan and set aside to cool.
2. Place a knife about an inch into your pork then insert garlic slivers, do this all over. Season pork using garlic powder, adobo, oregano, sazon and cumin. Pour chicken stock in your pot.
3. Stir in chipotle peppers and bay leaves then place pork in a deep pot. Cover and set to cook for 2 hours and 40 minutes over low heat.
4. Shred pork using forks and combine with juices. Remove bay leaves and mix well. Serve hot and enjoy.

NUTRITION: Calories 172 Fat 4.1g Protein 30.2g Carbs 2g

69. Slow Cooked Pork Tenderloin

Preparation Time: 5 minutes
Cooking time: 8 hours
Servings: 6
INGREDIENTS:

- 7 pounds of pork tenderloin
- ½ cup low sodium chicken broth
- 8 tbsp. stevia
- ½ tsp. garlic powder and cumin
- Salt and pepper for taste
- ¼ cup balsamic vinegar
- 9 tbsp. soy sauce
- ¼ tsp. chili powder

DIRECTIONS:
1. Add your soy sauce and vinegar to your slow cooker then stir to combine.
2. Add your remaining and spoon some of your vinegar mixture on top of the pork. Close the lid and allow to cook until very tender, usually about 6-8 hours.
3. If you want, you can reduce the cooking liquid to create a nice glaze. If you want a crisper outside, put it in a broiler for at least 4-5 minutes.

NUTRITION: Calories 264 Fat 6.4g Protein 40.6g Carbs 8.3g

70. Pork with Carrots & Apples

Preparation Time: 10 minutes
Cooking time: 10 minutes
Servings: 4
INGREDIENTS:

- 14 ½ boneless skinless pork loins (about ½ inch thick or 15 ounces each)
- 1 tablespoon of extra virgin olive oil, divided
- 1 teaspoon ground ginger
- ½ teaspoon ground sage
- ¼ teaspoon freshly ground black pepper
- 1 tablespoon unsalted fat free butter
- 1 large apple (Pink Lady works well), peeled, cored and cubed
- 1 cup diced carrots (approximately 5 16 small)
- ¼ cup water

DIRECTIONS:
1. Rub half the olive oil on all sides of pork. Mix ginger, sage, and pepper together and rub on both sides of pork chops.
2. Heat the other half of the oil in a large skillet over medium heat. Add pork to the skillet and sauté until brown, about 3 to 4 minutes per side and then transfer to a platter.

3. Add fat free butter, chopped apple, and carrots to the skillet and sauté until golden brown.
4. Stir in approximately ¼ cup of water and cook until tender. Add pork to the skillet and simmer until hot.

NUTRITION: Calories 337 Fat 6g Protein 33g Carbs 11g

71. Shredded Pork Tacos

Preparation Time: 10 minutes
Cooking time: 2 hours & 45 minutes
Servings: 11
INGREDIENTS:

- 17 ½ lbs. pork shoulder roast (trimmed, boneless)
- 6 garlic cloves (sliced)
- 1 ½ teaspoons cumin
- ¼ teaspoon oregano (dry)
- 18 teaspoons salt
- 19 bay leaves
- ¼ teaspoon adobo seasoning (dry)
- ½ teaspoon garlic powder
- 20 chipotle peppers (placed in adobo sauce)
- ½ teaspoon sazon
- Black pepper, to taste
- 1¾ cups chicken broth (reduced-sodium)
- Romaine lettuce leaves (enough to serve)

DIRECTIONS:
1. Season the pork with salt and pepper and brown it in a pot over medium heat for 5 minutes.
2. Using a knife out incisions on the pork and push garlic pieces in. Rub the oregano, adobo seasoning, cumin, sazon and garlic powder over the pork.
3. Replace the pork to the pot and add the rest of the ingredients. Cover and set to cook for 2 hours and 40 minutes on low heat or until fully cooked.
4. Shred the pork using forks and add back to the pot. Discard the bay leaves. Serve in warm Romaine lettuce leaves.

NUTRITION: Calories 130 Fat 7g Protein 20g Carbs 1g

72. Pork Ragu with Tagliatelle

Preparation Time: 5 minutes
Cooking time: 50 minutes
Servings: 4
INGREDIENTS:

- 9 oz. Tagliatelle
- 14 oz. extra lean minced pork

- 14 oz. tomatoes, chopped
- 21 garlic cloves, chopped
- 22 carrots, finely diced
- 23 celery sticks, chopped
- 1 finely chopped onion
- 24 tablespoons tomato puree
- 1 teaspoon olive oil
- ½ teaspoon dried oregano
- ½ teaspoon stevia
- 1 bay leaf
- 25 cups water
- Salt and pepper, to taste

DIRECTIONS:
1. Heat oil in a large non-stick frying pan, add minced pork and cook on a high heat for 5 minutes, stirring and breaking the meat up as it cooks.
2. Transfer cooked meat into a large saucepan, heat more olive oil in the frying pan and add carrots, onion and celery and cook over a low heat for 10 minutes, add a splash of water if required.
3. Stir in garlic and oregano and continue to cook for another 2 minutes, transfer the mixture into your saucepan. Add stevia, bay leaf and water.
4. Season with salt and pepper and bring to a boil, simmer for 45 minutes stirring occasionally until you have a rich and thick sauce.
5. Once your ragu is ready, cook pasta in accordance with the instructions on the packet and drain. Divide into bowls and top with sauce.

NUTRITION: Calories 363 Fat 8.9g Protein 25.7g Carbs 8.9g

73. Pork with Olives & Feta

Preparation Time: 10 minutes
Cooking time: 60 minutes
Servings: 4

INGREDIENTS:
- 26 lb. pork stew meat, cubed
- 30 oz spicy diced tomatoes with juice
- ½ cup black olives
- ½ cup green olives
- ½ tsp salt
- ¼ tsp black pepper
- 27 cups cooked rice

DIRECTIONS:
1. Put the pork, tomatoes, black olives and green olives in the Instant Pot. Season with salt and pepper.

2. Seal the pot. Turn to Manual. Cook on high for 1 hour. Top with the feta cheese. Serve with rice.

NUTRITION: Calories 378 Fat 9g Protein 36g Carbs 14g

74. Bone in Ham with Maple-Honey Glaze

Preparation Time: 5 minutes
Cooking time: 1 hour & 15 minutes
Servings: 14

INGREDIENTS:
- 8 tablespoons maple syrup
- 4 tablespoons honey
- 1½ cups orange juice
- 1 cup pineapple juice, sugar free
- 1 cinnamon sticks
- 1 bone-in ham

DIRECTIONS:
1. Create a glaze by combining your maple syrup, honey, orange juice, pineapple juice, and cinnamon together in a saucepan over medium heat. Mix well and allow to cook until the mixture thickens.
2. Remove from heat and set aside. Add your ham into a deep pot, cover and set to cook over medium heat for 50 minutes.
3. Transfer ham into oven safe dish and drizzle over glaze. Place under broiler till glaze is caramelized. Serve and enjoy.

NUTRITION: Calories 60 Fat 1g Protein 10g Carbs 3g

FISH PANCREATITIS DIET RECIPES

75. Scallop and Strawberry Salad

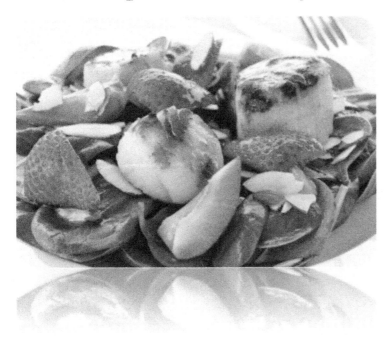

Preparation time: 2 hours
Cooking time: 6 minutes
Servings: 2

INGREDIENTS:

- 4 ounces scallops
- ½ cup Pico de gallo
- ½ cup chopped strawberries
- 1 tablespoon lime juice
- Salt and black pepper to the taste

DIRECTIONS:

1. Heat up a pan over medium heat, add scallops, cook for 3 minutes on each side and transfer to a bowl.
2. Add strawberries, lime juice, Pico de gallo, salt and pepper. Toss and serve cold after 2 hours. Enjoy!

NUTRITION: Calories 83 Fat 1g Carbs 5g Protein 14g

76. Halibut with Fruit Salad

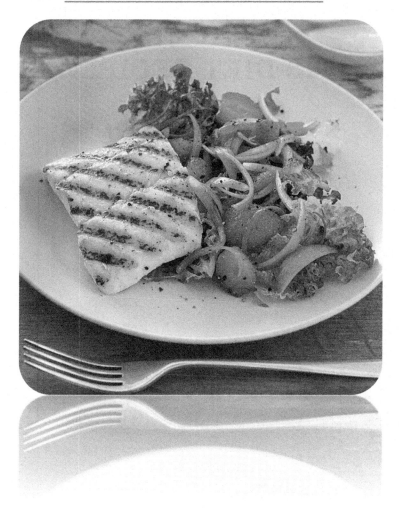

Preparation time: 10 minutes
Cooking time: 10 minutes
Servings: 4
INGREDIENTS:

- 4 halibut steaks, boneless
- 1 small cucumber, chopped
- 2 kiwis, peeled and chopped
- 3 cups strawberries, halved and then sliced
- 2 tablespoons olive oil
- Juice of ½ lemon
- A pinch of sea salt and black pepper
- A pinch of cayenne pepper
- ¼ teaspoon cinnamon powder
- 1/3 cup basil, chopped

- 6 cups micro greens

DIRECTIONS:

1. In a bowl, toss the cucumber with kiwi, strawberries, half of the oil, salt, pepper, basil, micro greens and lemon juice.
2. Season halibut steaks with salt, pepper, cinnamon and cayenne and drizzle with the rest of the oil then rub well.
3. Heat up a pan over medium-high heat, add the fish steaks, cook for 5 minutes on each side, divide between plates and serve with the fruity salad on the side. Enjoy!

NUTRITION: Calories 270 Fat 6g Carbs 13g Protein 15g

77. Poached Cod and Leeks

Preparation time: 10 minutes
Cooking time: 20 minutes
Servings: 4

INGREDIENTS:

- 4 cod fillets, skinless and boneless
- 2 cups veggie stock
- 2 tablespoons lemon juice
- 1 tablespoon fresh grated ginger
- 4 teaspoons lemon zest
- A pinch of sea salt and black pepper
- 3 leeks, chopped
- 2 tablespoons olive oil
- 1 pound kale, chopped
- ½ teaspoon sesame oil

DIRECTIONS:

1. In a bowl, mix lemon zest with salt and pepper then stir and rub the fish with this mix. Heat up a pan with the stock over medium heat.
2. Add leeks, ginger and lemon juice then stir, bring to a simmer, and cook for a few minutes. Add fish fillets to this mix, cover pan, poach the fish for 10 minutes, transfer it to a dish, strain the liquid and reserve the leeks.
3. Heat up a pan with the olive oil over medium heat and add kale then cook for 3-4 minutes. Add strained soup and cook for 5 minutes more.
4. Add reserved leeks, stir, cook for 2 minutes more and take off heat. Divide fish into bowls and top each fillet with the leek soup. Drizzle the sesame oil all over and serve. Enjoy!

NUTRITION: Calories 278 Fat 3g Carbs 14g Protein 15g

78. Cilantro Halibut with Coconut Milk

Preparation time: 10 minutes
Cooking time: 10 minutes
Servings: 4

INGREDIENTS:

- ¼ cup coconut milk
- ¼ cup chopped cilantro
- 1 tablespoon green curry paste
- ¼ cup chopped basil
- 2 teaspoons coconut aminos
- ½ teaspoon ground turmeric
- 4 halibut fillets, boneless
- 1 tablespoon avocado oil
- 1 red chili pepper, chopped

DIRECTIONS:

1. In your blender, puree the cilantro with coconut milk, chili pepper, basil, aminos, curry paste and turmeric.
2. Heat up a pan with the oil over medium-high heat, add halibut fillets and cook for 4 minutes on each side.
3. Add the coconut mix over the fish and toss gently/ Cook for 2 minutes more, divide everything between plates and serve. Enjoy!

NUTRITION: Calories 210 Fat 3g Carbs 12g Protein 16

79. Easy Baked Cod

Preparation time: 10 minutes
Cooking time: 12 minutes
Servings: 2

INGREDIENTS:

- 2 cod fillets, boneless
- 1 garlic cloves, minced
- 1 teaspoon olive oil
- Black pepper to the taste
- 3 sun-dried tomatoes, chopped
- 1 small red onion, sliced
- ½ fennel bulb, thinly sliced
- 4 black olives, pitted and sliced
- 2 rosemary springs
- ¼ teaspoon red pepper flakes

DIRECTIONS:

1. Grease a baking dish with the oil, add the cod, garlic, black pepper, tomatoes, onion, fennel, olives, rosemary and pepper flakes.
2. Cover the dish, bake at 400 degrees F for 14 minutes then discard the rosemary, divide the fish and veggies between plates and serve. Enjoy!

NUTRITION: Calories 260 Fat 4g Carbs 10g Protein 16g

80. Herbed Salmon with Onions

Preparation time: 10 minutes
Cooking time: 30 minutes
Servings: 2

INGREDIENTS:

- 16 ounces pearl onions
- A drizzle of olive oil
- 2 medium salmon fillets, boneless
- 1 tablespoon dried parsley
- 1 teaspoon dried rosemary
- Black pepper to the taste

DIRECTIONS:

1. Put the salmon in a baking dish, add the oil, parsley, rosemary and black pepper. Toss a bit, bake in the oven at 375 degrees F for 30 minutes, divide between plates and serve. Enjoy!

NUTRITION: Calories 260 Fat 3g Carbs 7g Protein 16g

81. Chinese Salmon

Preparation time: 10 minutes
Cooking time: 10 minutes
Servings: 2

INGREDIENTS:

- 2 salmon steaks
- 4 tablespoons chopped green onions
- 4 tablespoons coconut aminos
- 2 garlic cloves, minced
- 2 tablespoons olive oil
- 1 teaspoon saffron powder

DIRECTIONS:

1. In a bowl, whisk the green onions with aminos, garlic, oil and saffron. Add the salmon steaks, toss them well, place them on the preheated grill over medium heat.
2. Cook for 5 minutes on each side. Divide between plates and serve with a side salad. Enjoy!

NUTRITION: Calories 251 Fat 8g Carbs 13g Protein 16g

82. Spinach and Scallop

Preparation time: 10 minutes
Cooking time: 10 minutes
Servings: 4

INGREDIENTS:

- 12 jumbo sea scallops

- A pinch of sea salt and black pepper
- A drizzle of olive oil
- 6 garlic cloves, minced
- 1 cup chopped yellow onion
- 12 ounces baby spinach

DIRECTIONS:
1. Heat up the pan with the oil over medium heat then add scallops, season with salt and black pepper and cook for 3 minutes on each side then divide between plates.
2. Heat up the pan again over medium heat, add garlic and onions, stir and cook for 3 minutes. Add spinach, toss, cook for 3 minutes more and serve next to the scallops. Enjoy!

NUTRITION: Calories 206 Fat 6g Carbs 7g Protein 17g

83. Crab Salad

Preparation time: 10 minutes
Cooking time: 0 minutes
Servings: 3

INGREDIENTS:
- 2 cups avocado, peeled, pitted and cubed
- 1 cup chopped cucumber
- 2 cups canned crab, drained and flaked
- 2 teaspoons chopped parsley
- A pinch of salt and black pepper
- ½ tablespoon olive oil
- 1 tablespoon lime juice

DIRECTIONS:
1. In a salad bowl, mix the avocado with crab, cucumber, parsley, salt, pepper, oil and lime juice. Toss well and serve. Enjoy!

NUTRITION: Calories 260 Fat 17g Carbs 11g Protein 18g

84. Garlic Cod Soup

Preparation time: 2 hours
Cooking time: 20 minutes
Servings: 4

INGREDIENTS:
- 2 pounds cod fillets, cubed
- 10 garlic cloves, minced
- 3 tablespoons olive oil
- 1 tablespoon lemon juice
- ¼ cup chopped parsley
- 1 yellow onion, chopped

- 2 tomatoes, chopped
- 1 tablespoon tomato paste
- 2 ½ cups veggie stock
- A pinch of sea salt and black pepper
- 10 cherry tomatoes, halved

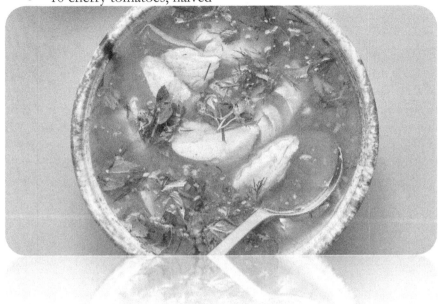

DIRECTIONS:
1. In a bowl, mix 6 garlic cloves with 2 tablespoons oil, parsley, lemon juice and the fish. Toss the fish to coat then cover bowl and keep in the fridge for 2 hours to marinate.
2. Heat up a pot with the rest of the oil over medium-high heat, add onion, stir and cook for 2 minutes.
3. Add the rest of the garlic, tomatoes, tomato paste, stock, salt, pepper and marinated fish and mix. Bring to a simmer and cook for 10 minutes.
4. Add cherry tomatoes, stir, cook for 6 minutes more, ladle soup into bowls and serve. Enjoy!

NUTRITION: Calories 160 Fat 2g Carbs 4g Protein 7g

85. Chili Coconut Salmon

Preparation time: 10 minutes
Cooking time: 15 minutes
Servings: 6
INGREDIENTS:
- 1 ¼ cups shredded coconut, unsweetened
- 1 pound salmon, cubed
- 1/3 cup coconut flour
- A pinch of salt and black pepper

- 1 egg
- 2 tablespoons olive oil
- ¼ cup water
- 4 red chilies, chopped
- 3 garlic cloves, minced
- ¼ cup balsamic vinegar
- ½ cup raw honey

DIRECTIONS:
1. In a bowl, mix coconut flour with a pinch of salt and stir. In another bowl, whisk the egg with black pepper and put the shredded coconut in a third bowl.
2. Dip salmon cubes in the coconut flour then in the egg and then in the shredded coconut mix. Heat up a pan with the oil over medium-high heat, add salmon and fry for 3 minutes on each side then divide between plates.
3. Heat up a pan with the water over medium-high heat, add chilies, cloves, vinegar and honey. Stir, bring to a gentle boil, simmer for 4 minutes then drizzle over the salmon and serve. Enjoy!

NUTRITION: Calories 211 Fat 5g Carbs 11g Protein 15

86. Clams with Olives Mix

Preparation time: 10 minutes
Cooking time: 10 minutes
Servings: 2

INGREDIENTS:
- 3 tablespoons olive oil
- 2-pound little clams, scrubbed
- ½ teaspoon dried thyme
- 1 shallot, minced
- ½ cup veggie stock
- 2 garlic cloves, minced
- 1 apple, cored and chopped
- Juice of ½ lemon

DIRECTIONS:
1. Heat up a pan with the oil over medium-high heat, add shallot and garlic, stir and cook for 3-4 minutes.
2. Add the stock, clams, thyme, apple and lemon juice. Stir and cook for 6 minutes more, divide into bowls and serve. Enjoy!

NUTRITION: Calories 180 Fat 9g Carbs 8g Protein 10g

87. Classy Soup with Carrot and Ginger

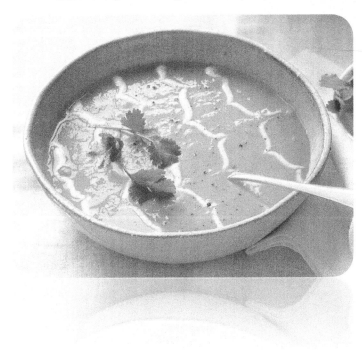

Preparation Time: 10 minutes
Cooking time: 30 minutes
Servings: 6-8

INGREDIENTS:
- 1 large onion, peeled and roughly chopped
- 4½ cups plus 2 tablespoons water, divided
- 8 carrots, peeled and roughly chopped
- 1½-inch piece thin fresh ginger, sliced
- 1¼ teaspoons sea salt
- 2 cups coconut milk, unsweetened

DIRECTIONS:
1. Sauté the onion in 2 tablespoons of water for about 5 minutes, or until soft in a large pot set over medium heat.
2. Add the carrots, the remaining 4½ cups of water, the ginger, and salt. Bring to a boil. Reduce the heat to low and cover the pot. Simmer for 20 minutes.
3. Stir in the coconut milk and for 4 to 5 minutes, let it heat. Blend the soup in a blender until creamy, working in batches if necessary and taking care of the hot liquid.

NUTRITION: Calories: 228 Fat: 19g Carbs: 15g Protein: 3g

88. Creamy Soup with Broccoli

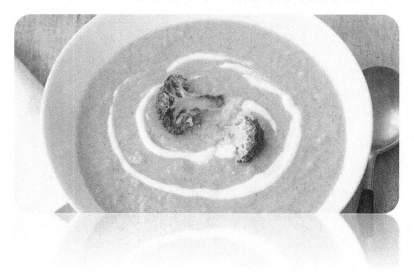

Preparation Time: 12 minutes
Cooking time: 25 minutes
Servings: 6

INGREDIENTS:

- 1 onion, finely chopped
- 4 garlic cloves, finely chopped
- 5 cups plus 2 tablespoons water, divided
- 1½ teaspoons sea salt, plus additional as needed
- 4 broccoli heads with stalks, heads cut into florets, and stalks roughly chopped
- 1 cup cashews, soaked in water for 4 hours

DIRECTIONS:

1. Sauté the onion and garlic in 2 tablespoons of water in a large pot set over medium heat for about 5 minutes, or until soft.
2. Add the remaining 5 cups of water, salt, and broccoli. Bring to a boil. Cover and reduce the heat to low. Simmer for 20 minutes.
3. Drain and rinse the cashews. Transfer them to a blender.
4. Add the soup to the blender. Blend until smooth, working in batches if necessary, and taking care of the hot liquid. Taste, and adjust the seasoning if necessary.

NUTRITION: Calories: 224 Fat: 11g Carbs: 26g Protein: 11g

89. Classic Soup with Butternut Squash

Preparation Time: 20 minutes
Cooking time: 30 minutes
Servings: 6

INGREDIENTS:

- 1 onion, chopped roughly

- 4½ cups plus 2 tablespoons water, divided
- 1 large butternut squash, washed, peeled, ends trimmed, halved, seeded, and cut into ½-inch chunks
- 2 celery stalks, chopped roughly
- 3 carrots, peeled and chopped roughly
- 1 teaspoon sea salt, plus additional as needed

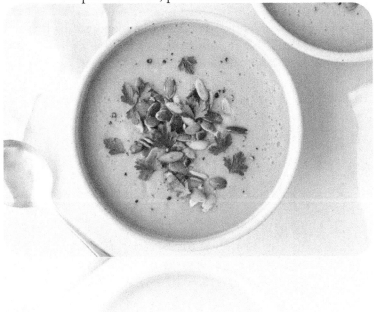

DIRECTIONS:
1. Sauté the onion in 2 tablespoons of water in a large pot set over medium heat for about 5 minutes, or until soft.
2. Add the squash, celery, carrot, and salt. Bring to a boil. Reduce the heat to low, Cover, and simmer for 25 minutes.
3. Purée the soup in a blender until smooth, working in batches if necessary and taking care of the hot liquid. Taste, and adjust the seasoning if necessary.

NUTRITION: Calories: 104 Carbs: 27g Fat: 0g Protein: 2g

90. Thai Soup with Potato

Preparation Time: 10 minutes
Cooking time: 20-25 minutes
Servings: 4-6
INGREDIENTS:
- 3 large sweet potatoes, cubed
- 2 cups water
- One 14 ounces can coconut milk
- ½-inch piece fresh ginger, sliced

- ½ cup almond butter
- Zest of 1 lime
- Juice of 1 lime
- 1 teaspoon salt, plus additional as needed

DIRECTIONS:
1. Combine the sweet potatoes, water, coconut milk, and ginger in a large pot set over high heat. Bring to a boil. Reduce the heat to low and cover.
2. For 20 to 25 minutes, simmer until the potatoes are tender. Transfer to a blender the potatoes, ginger, and cooking liquid.
3. Add the almond butter, lime zest, lime juice, and salt. Blend until smooth. Taste, and adjust the seasoning if necessary.

NUTRITION: Calories: 653 Fat: 42g Carbs: 64g Protein: 12g

91. Extraordinary Creamy Green Soup

Preparation Time: 10 minutes
Cooking time: 15 minutes
Servings: 4-6

INGREDIENTS:
- 3 cups water
- 2 cups coconut milk, unsweetened
- 1½ teaspoons sea salt, plus additional as needed
- 4 cups tightly packed kale, washed thoroughly, stemmed, and roughly chopped
- 4 cups tightly packed spinach, stemmed and roughly chopped
- 4 cups tightly packed collard greens, stemmed and roughly chopped
- 1 bunch fresh parsley, stemmed and roughly chopped

DIRECTIONS:
1. Bring the water, coconut milk, and salt to a boil in a large pot set over high heat. Reduce the heat to low.
2. Add the kale, spinach, and collard greens 1 cup at a time then let them wilt before adding the next cup. Continue until all the greens have been added to the pot.
3. For 8 to 10 minutes, simmer. Blend the soup in a blender until smooth, working in batches if necessary and taking care of the hot liquid. Taste, and adjust the seasoning before serving.

NUTRITION: Calories: 334 Fat: 29g Carbs: 18g Protein: 7g

92. Zingy Soup with Ginger, Carrot, and Lime

Preparation Time: 5 minutes
Cooking time: 40 minutes
Servings: 2

INGREDIENTS:
- 2 tablespoon olive oil
- 1 teaspoon mustard seeds, ground

- 1 teaspoon coriander seeds, ground
- 1 teaspoon curry powder
- 1 teaspoon ginger, minced
- 4 cups carrots, thinly sliced
- 2 cups onions, chopped
- zest and juice of 1 lime
- 4 cups low-salt vegetable broth
- black pepper

DIRECTIONS:
1. Heat the oil in a pan on medium heat and for 1 minute, add the seeds and curry powder. Add the ginger and then cook for another minute.
2. Then add in the carrots, onions, and the lime zest, cooking for at least 2 minutes or until the vegetables are soft.
3. Add the broth and allow to boil before turning the heat down slightly and allowing to simmer for 30 minutes.
4. Allow cooling. Put the mixture in a food processor and purée until smooth. Serve with lime juice and black pepper.

NUTRITION: Calories: 919 Fat: 51g Carbs: 105g Protein: 13g

93. Native Asian Soup with Squash and Shitake

Preparation Time: 10 minutes
Cooking time: 45 minutes
Servings: 2

INGREDIENTS:
- 15 dried shiitake mushrooms, soaked in water
- 6 cups low salt vegetable stock
- ½ butternut squash, peeled and cubed
- 1 tablespoon sesame oil
- 1 onion, quartered and sliced into rings
- 1 large garlic clove, chopped
- 4 stems of pak choy or equivalent
- 1 sprig of thyme or 1 tablespoon dried thyme
- 1 teaspoon tabasco sauce

DIRECTIONS:
1. Heat sesame on medium-high heat oil in a large pan before sweating the onions and garlic. Add the vegetable stock and bring to a boil over a high heat before adding the squash.
2. Turn down the heat and allow to simmer for 25 to 30 minutes. Soak the mushrooms in the water if not already done, and then press out the liquid and add to the stock into the pot.
3. Use the mushroom water in the stock for extra taste. Except for the greens, add the rest of the ingredients and allow to simmer for 15 minutes more or until the squash is tender.

4. Before serving, add in the chopped greens and let them wilt. Serve with the tabasco sauce if you like it spicy.

NUTRITION: Calories: 1191 Fat: 56g Carbs: 158g Protein: 19g

94. Peppery Soup with Tomato

Preparation Time: 2 minutes
Cooking time: 35 minutes
Servings: 2

INGREDIENTS:
- 2 red bell peppers
- 4 beef tomatoes
- 1 sweet onion, chopped
- 1 garlic clove, chopped
- 3 cups homemade chicken broth
- 2 habanero chilis, stems removed and chopped
- 2 tablespoon extra-virgin olive oil

DIRECTIONS:
1. Preheat the broiler to medium-high heat and grill the bell peppers, turning halfway for 10 minutes until the skins are blackened.
2. Heat water in a pan on medium to high heat and cut a small x at the bottom of each tomato using a sharp knife.
3. Transfer to separate dish pepper once cooked and cover. For 20 seconds, blanch the tomatoes in simmering water.
4. Remove and plunge into ice-cold water. Peel and chop tomatoes, reserving the juices.
5. Sauté the onion, garlic, chili, and 2 tablespoons of oil in a saucepan on medium-high heat, stirring for 8-10 minutes until golden.
6. Add the tomatoes with the juices, the peppers, and broth to the onions and cover and simmer for 10-15 minutes or until heated through. Purée in a blender and serve.

NUTRITION: Calories: 741 Fat: 32g Carbs: 30g Protein: 82g

95. Moroccan Inspired Lentil Soup

Preparation Time: 5 minutes
Cooking time: 40 minutes
Servings: 2

INGREDIENTS:
- 2 tablespoon extra-virgin olive oil
- 1 yellow onion, diced
- 1 carrot, diced
- 1 clove of minced garlic, diced
- 1 teaspoon cumin, ground
- ½ teaspoon ginger, ground

- 2 tablespoon low-fat Greek yogurt
- ½ teaspoon turmeric, ground
- ½ teaspoon red chili flakes
- 1 can tomatoes, chopped
- 1 cup dried yellow lentils, soaked
- 5 cups of low salt vegetable stock or homemade chicken stock
- 1 lemon

DIRECTIONS:
1. Heat the oil in a large pan on medium-high heat. Sauté the onion and carrot for 5 to 6 minutes until softened and starting to brown.
2. Add the garlic, ginger, chili flakes, cumin, and turmeric, cook for 2 minutes.
3. Add the tomatoes, scraping any brown bits from the bottom of the pan, and cooking until the liquid is reduced for 15 to 20 minutes).
4. Add the lentils and stock and turn the heat up to reach a boil before lowering the heat, covering, and for 10 minutes, simmer.
5. Serve with a wedge of lemon on the side and a dollop of Greek yogurt.

NUTRITION: Calories: 1048 Fat: 53g Carbs: 128g Protein: 19g

96. Classic Vegetarian Tagine

Preparation Time: 10 minutes
Cooking time: 45 minutes
Servings: 2

INGREDIENTS:
- 2 tablespoon coconut oil
- 1 onion, diced
- 1 parsnip, peeled and diced
- 2 cloves of garlic
- 1 teaspoon cumin, ground
- ½ teaspoon ginger, ground
- ½ teaspoon cinnamon, ground
- ¼ teaspoon cayenne pepper
- 3 tablespoon tomato paste
- 1 sweet potato, peeled & diced
- 1 purple potato, peeled & diced
- 4 baby carrots, peeled & diced
- 4 cups low-salt vegetable stock
- 2 cups kale leaves
- 2 tablespoons lemon juice
- ¼ cup cilantro, roughly chopped
- handful of almonds, toasted

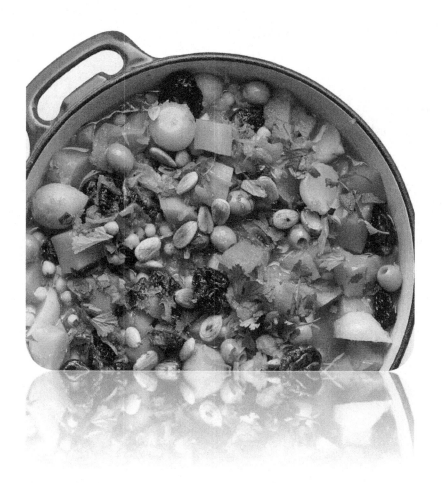

DIRECTIONS:
1. Heat the oil in a large pot on a medium-high heat before sautéing the onion until soft. Add the parsnip for 10 minutes or until golden brown.
2. Add the garlic, cumin, ginger, cinnamon, tomato paste, and cayenne. For 2 minutes, cook until it has a lovely scent.
3. Fold in the sweet potatoes, carrots, and purple potatoes and stock and then bring to a boil. Turn heat down and simmer for 20 minutes.
4. Add in the kale and lemon juice, simmering for 2 minutes more or until the leaves are slightly wilted. Garnish with cilantro and the nuts to serve.

NUTRITION: Calories: 1115 Fat: 51g Carbs: 150g Protein: 19g

97. Homemade Warm and Chunky Chicken Soup

Preparation Time: 7 minutes
Cooking time: 40 minutes
Servings: 4
INGREDIENTS:
- 1 whole free-range chicken, cooked and no giblets
- 1 bay leaf

- 5 cups of homemade chicken broth/water
- 1 onion, chopped
- 2 stalks of celery, sliced
- 3 carrots, chopped and peeled
- 2 parsnips, chopped and peeled
- sprinkle of pepper

DIRECTIONS:
1. Into a large pot, add all of the ingredients minus the pepper, and boil on high heat. Lower the heat once boiling and allow to simmer for 30 minutes, or until the chicken is piping hot.
2. Remove the chicken and place it on a chopping board. Slice as much meat as you can from the chicken and remove the skin and bones.
3. Add it back into the pot and either serve right away as a chunky soup or allow it to cool and whizz through the blender to serve.
4. Add black pepper to season and serve alone or with your choice of whole-grain bread, just pop it into the soup 20 minutes before the end to soak up all the delicious flavors.

NUTRITION: Calories: 101 Fat: 1g Carbs: 22g Protein: 7g

98. Indian Curried Stew with Lentil and Spinach

Preparation Time: 5 minutes
Cooking time: 30 minutes
Servings: 2

INGREDIENTS:
- 1 tablespoon extra-virgin olive oil
- 1 tablespoon curry powder
- 1 cup homemade chicken or vegetable stock
- 1 cup red lentils, soaked
- 1 onion, chopped
- 2 cups butternut squash, cooked peeled, and chopped
- 1 cup spinach
- 2 garlic cloves, minced
- 1 tablespoon cilantro, finely chopped

DIRECTIONS:
1. Add the oil, chopped onion, and minced garlic, sauté for 5 minutes on low heat in a large pot. Add the curry powder and ginger to the onions and cook for 5 minutes.
2. Add the broth and bring to a boil on high heat. Stir in the lentils, squash, and spinach, reduce heat and simmer for 20 minutes more.
3. Season with pepper to taste and serve with fresh cilantro.

NUTRITION: Calories: 1022 Fat: 19g Carbs: 91g Protein: 123g

99. Soulful Roasted Vegetable Soup

Preparation Time: 10 minutes

Cooking time: 30 minutes
Servings: 2
INGREDIENTS:

- 2 medium carrots, peeled
- 1 cup baby Brussels sprouts
- 1 rib celery
- ¼ medium head cabbage
- 2 teaspoons fine Himalayan salt, divided
- 2 tablespoons coconut oil
- 2 cups bone broth
- ½ medium Hass avocado, peeled, pitted, and sliced
- 1 green onion, minced
- 4 sprigs fresh cilantro, minced

DIRECTIONS:

1. Preheat the oven to 400°F.
2. Cut all of the vegetables into small pieces and spread them out on a sheet pan. Sprinkle with 1 teaspoon of the salt and toss with the coconut oil. For 30 minutes, roast.
3. Heat the broth in a saucepan while the vegetables are roasting over medium heat.
4. Divide the vegetables between two serving bowls when they are ready. Add the avocado, green onion, and cilantro, and sprinkle in the remaining teaspoon of salt. Divide the broth between the bowls.
5. Serve immediately. Store leftovers in an airtight container in the fridge for up to 4 days.

NUTRITION: Calories: 276 Fat: 23g Carbs: 19gProtein: 6g

100.   Corn Chowder

Preparation Time: 20 minutes
Cooking time: 50 minutes
Servings: 4
INGREDIENTS:

- 3 tablespoons avocado oil
- 2 cups onions, diced
- 3 cups bone broth
- 2 cups cauliflower pearls
- ¾ cup coconut cream
- 2 teaspoons black pepper, ground
- 1 teaspoon fine Himalayan salt
- ½ teaspoon cumin, ground
- ½ teaspoon nutmeg, ground
- 2 tablespoons nutritional yeast
- Leaves from fresh thyme sprig
- 2 tablespoons Garlic Confit

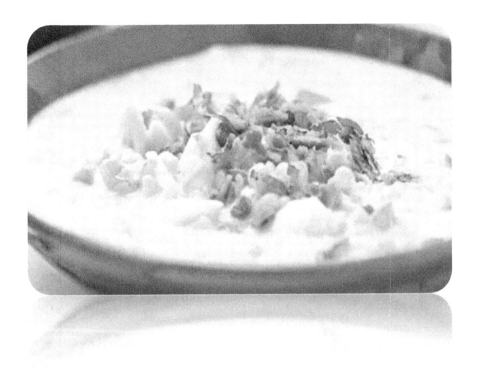

DIRECTIONS:

1. Place a medium-sized pot over medium heat. Pour in the avocado oil and add the diced onion when it's hot. Lower the heat to medium-low and cover.
2. For 20 minutes, cook and stir once halfway through. The onions should be browned but not crispy since they need to be soft and sweet.
3. Add the broth, cauliflower, coconut cream, and seasonings. Stir well and bring to a simmer. For 20 to 30 minutes, simmer and stir occasionally.
4. It's time to make it creamy when the soup has reduced by one-third and the chunks of onion and cauliflower protrude through the broth.
5. Into a blender, pour half of the soup. Make sure you're not just pouring out broth; you want to get plenty of cauliflower and onion into the blender, too.
6. Blend until silky smooth, then pour the purée back into the pot and stir to combine it all, creating a creamy soup studded with tender pearls of cauliflower and sweet onion.
7. Garnish with the thyme and garlic confit before serving. Store leftovers in an airtight container in the fridge for up to 5 days or in the freezer for up to 30 days. Bring to a simmer on the stovetop to reheat.

NUTRITION: Calories: 202 Fat: 13g Carbs: 14g Protein: 12g

101. Egg Drop Soup

Preparation Time: 5 minutes
Cooking time: 25 minutes
Servings: 4

INGREDIENTS:

- 2 tablespoons sesame oil, toasted

- 2-inch piece fresh ginger, peeled
- 4 cloves garlic, peeled
- 4 cups bone broth
- 1 tablespoon coconut aminos
- 1 tablespoon fish sauce
- Pinch of fine Himalayan salt
- 4 large eggs, whisked
- 2 green onions, sliced,
- 4 sprigs fresh cilantro, minced,

DIRECTIONS:

1. Heat the sesame oil in a 6- or 8-quart pot over medium heat. Add the ginger and garlic and stir until lightly browned.
2. Add the broth, coconut aminos, fish sauce, and salt. Bring to a low simmer, reduce the heat to low, cover, and cook for 20 minutes.
3. Slowly drizzle in the eggs while stirring the soup so the eggs cook instantly in ribbons as they hit the broth.
4. Garnish with green onions and cilantro and serve hot. Store leftovers in an airtight container in the fridge for up to 5 days.

NUTRITION: Calories: 185 Fat: 12g Carbs: 4g Protein: 16g

102. Okra Fries

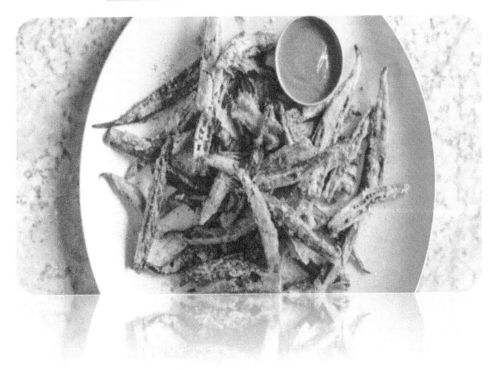

Preparation time: 15 minutes
Cooking time: 35 minutes
Servings: 4

INGREDIENTS:

- 2 tablespoons olive oil, divided
- 3 tablespoons creole seasoning
- ½ teaspoon ground turmeric
- 1 teaspoon water
- 1-pound okra, trimmed and slit in the middle

DIRECTIONS:

1. Preheat the oven at 450 degrees F. Line a baking sheet that has foil paper and grease with 1 tablespoon of oil.
2. In a bowl, mix creole seasoning, turmeric, and water. Fill the slits of okra with turmeric mixture.
3. Place the okra onto a prepared baking sheet in a very single layer. Bake for around 30-35 minutes, flipping once inside the middle way.

NUTRITION: Calories: 119 Fat: 6.98g Carbohydrates: 12.43g Protein: 2.51g

103. Potato Sticks

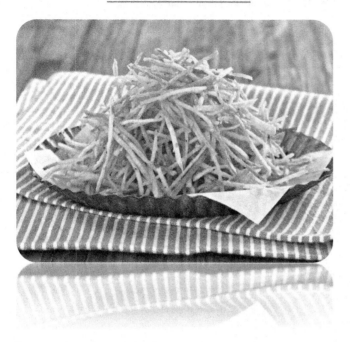

Preparation time: 15 minutes
Cooking time: 10 minutes
Servings: 2

INGREDIENTS:

- 1 large russet potato, peeled and cut into 1/8-inch thick sticks lengthwise
- 10 curry leaves
- ¼ teaspoon ground turmeric
- ¼ teaspoon red chili powder
- Salt, to taste
- 1 tbsp essential olive oil

DIRECTIONS:

1. Preheat the oven at 400 degrees F. Line 2 baking sheets with parchment papers.
2. In a sizable bowl, add all ingredients and toss to coat well. Transfer the amalgamation into prepared baking sheets in a single layer.
3. Bake for around 10 minutes. Serve immediately.

NUTRITION: Calories: 175 Fat: 3.21g Carbohydrates: 33.78g Protein: 4.06g

104. Zucchini Chips

Preparation time: 15 minutes
Cooking time: 15 minutes
Servings: 2

INGREDIENTS:

- 1 medium zucchini, cut into thin slices

- 1/8 teaspoon ground turmeric
- 1/8 teaspoon ground cumin
- Salt, to taste
- 2 teaspoons essential olive oil

DIRECTIONS:
1. Preheat the oven at 400 degrees F. Line 2 baking sheets with parchment papers.
2. In a substantial bowl, add all ingredients and toss to coat well. Transfer a combination into prepared baking sheets in a single layer.
3. Bake approximately 10-fifteen minutes. Serve immediately.

NUTRITION: Calories: 20 Fat: 2g Carbohydrates: 0.37g Protein: 0.21g

105.   Beet Chips

Preparation time: 15 minutes
Cooking time: 20 minutes
Servings: 2

INGREDIENTS:
- 1 beetroot, trimmed, peeled, and sliced thinly
- 1 teaspoon garlic, minced
- 1 tablespoon nutritional yeast
- ½ teaspoon red chili powder
- 2 teaspoons coconut oil, melted

DIRECTIONS:
1. Preheat the oven at 375 degrees F. Line a baking sheet using parchment paper.
2. In a large bowl, add all ingredients and toss to coat well.
3. Transfer the mixture into a prepared baking sheet in a very single layer.
4. Bake approximately twenty minutes, flipping once inside the middle way. Serve immediately.

NUTRITION: Calories: 80 Fat: 4.5g Carbohydrates: 6g Protein: 3g

106.   Spinach Chips

Preparation time: 10 minutes
Cooking time: 8 minutes
Servings: 1

INGREDIENTS:
- 2 cups fresh spinach leaves
- Few drops of extra-virgin olive oil
- Salt, to taste
- Italian seasoning, to taste

DIRECTIONS:
1. Preheat the oven at 325 degrees F. Line a baking sheet with parchment paper.
2. In a substantial bowl, add spinach leaves and drizzle with oil. With the hands, rub the spinach leaves till the leaves are coated with oil.

3. Transfer the leaves into a prepared baking sheet in a very single layer. Bake for about 8 minutes. Serve immediately.

NUTRITION: Calories: 14 Fat: 4.5g Carbohydrates: 2.18g Protein: 1.72g

107. Sweet & Tangy Seeds Crackers

Preparation time: 15 minutes
Cooking time: 12 hours
Servings: 10
INGREDIENTS:
- 2 cups water
- 1 cup sunflower seeds
- 1 cup flaxseeds
- 1 tablespoon fresh ginger, chopped
- 1 teaspoon raw honey
- ¼ cup freshly squeezed lemon juice
- 1 teaspoon ground turmeric
- Salt, to taste

DIRECTIONS:
1. In a bowl, add water, sunflower seeds, and flaxseeds and soak for around overnight. Drain the seeds.
2. In a food processor, add soaked seeds and remaining ingredients and pulse till well combined. Set dehydrator at 115 degrees F. Line a dehydrator tray with unbleached parchment paper.
3. Place the mix onto the prepared dehydrator tray evenly. With a knife, score how big crackers. Dehydrate for about 12 hours.

NUTRITION: Calories: 176 Fat: 14.32g Carbohydrates: 8.97g Protein: 6.05g

108. Plantain Chips

Preparation time: quarter-hour
Cooking time: 10 min
Servings: 1
INGREDIENTS:
- 1 plantain, peeled and sliced
- ½ teaspoon ground turmeric
- Salt, to taste
- 1 teaspoon coconut oil, melted

DIRECTIONS:
1. In a large bowl, add all ingredients and toss to coat well. Transfer the half in the mixture in a large greased bowl. Microwave on high for around 3 minutes.
2. Now, decrease the capacity to 50% and microwave for approximately 2 minutes. Repeat with the remaining plantain mixture.

NUTRITION: Calories: 222 Fat: 4.83g Carbohydrates: 48.98g Protein: 1.36g

109. Quinoa & Seeds Crackers

Preparation time: 15 minutes
Cooking time: 20 or so minutes
Servings: 6
INGREDIENTS:

- 3 tablespoons water
- 1 tablespoon chia seeds
- 3 tablespoons sunflower seeds
- 1 tablespoon quinoa flour
- 1 teaspoon ground turmeric
- Pinch of ground cinnamon
- Salt, to taste

DIRECTIONS:
1. Preheat the oven at 345 degrees F. Line a baking sheet with parchment paper.
2. In a bowl, add water and chia seeds and soak for approximately a quarter-hour.
3. After fifteen minutes, add the remaining ingredients and mix well.
4. Spread the mix onto a prepared baking sheet. Bake approximately 20 minutes.

NUTRITION: Calories: 34 Fat: 2.38g Carbohydrates: 2.35g Protein: 1.21g

110. Apple Leather

Preparation time: 15 minutes
Cooking time: 12 hours, 25 minutes
Servings: 4
INGREDIENTS:

- 1 cup water
- 8 cups apples, peeled, cored, and chopped
- 1 tablespoon ground cinnamon
- 2 tablespoons freshly squeezed lemon juice

DIRECTIONS:
1. In a big pan, add water and apples on medium-low heat. Simmer, stirring occasionally for around 10-quarter-hour. Remove from heat and make aside to cool slightly.
2. In a blender, add apple mixture and pulse till smooth. Return the mixture into the pan on medium-low heat.
3. Stir in cinnamon and fresh lemon juice and simmer for approximately 10 minutes. Transfer the mix onto dehydrator trays and with the back of the spoon smooth the very best.
4. Set the dehydrator at 135 degrees F. Dehydrate for around 10-12 hours. Cut the apple leather into equal-sized rectangles. Now, roll each rectangle to make fruit rolls.

NUTRITION: Calories: 120 Fat: 0.41g Carbohydrates: 32.2g Protein: 0.67g

111.   Roasted Cashews

Preparation time: 5 minutes
Cooking time: 20 or so minutes
Servings: 16

INGREDIENTS:

- 2 cups cashews
- 2 teaspoons raw honey
- 1½ teaspoons smoked paprika
- ½ teaspoon chili flakes
- Salt, to taste
- 1 tablespoon freshly squeezed lemon juice
- 1 teaspoon organic olive oil

DIRECTIONS:

1. Preheat the oven at 350 degrees F. Line a baking dish with parchment paper. In a bowl, add all ingredients and toss to coat well.
2. Transfer the cashew mixture into a baking dish inside a single layer. Roast for approximately 20 min, flipping once inside the middle way.
3. Remove from oven and make aside to cool before serving. You can preserve these roasted cashews in an airtight jar.

NUTRITION: Calories: 200 Fat: 17.13g Carbohydrates: 10.65g Protein: 3.93g

112.   Roasted Pumpkin Seeds

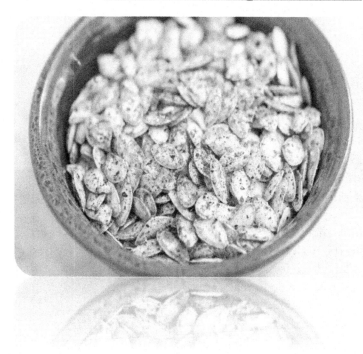

Preparation time: 10 minutes
Cooking time: 20 minutes
Servings: 4

INGREDIENTS:

- 1 cup pumpkin seeds, washed and dried
- 2 teaspoons garam masala
- 1/3 teaspoon red chili powder
- ¼ teaspoon ground turmeric
- Salt, to taste
- 3 tablespoons coconut oil, melted
- ½ tablespoon fresh lemon juice

DIRECTIONS:

1. Preheat the oven at 350 degrees F. In a bowl, add all ingredients except lemon juice and toss to coat well.
2. Transfer the almond mixture right into a baking sheet. Roast approximately twenty or so minutes, flipping occasionally.
3. Remove from oven and make aside to cool before serving. Drizzle with freshly squeezed lemon juice and serve.

NUTRITION: Calories: 259 Fat: 24.71g Carbohydrates: 4.72g Protein: 8.86g

113. Spiced Popcorn

Preparation time: 5 minutes
Cooking time: 2 minutes
Servings: 2-3

INGREDIENTS:

- 3 tablespoons coconut oil
- ½ cup popping corn
- 1 tbsp olive oil
- 1 teaspoon ground turmeric
- ¼ teaspoon garlic
- Salt, to taste

DIRECTIONS:

1. In a pan, melt coconut oil on medium-high heat. Add popping corn and cover the pan tightly.
2. Cook, shaking the pan occasionally for around 1-2 minutes or till corn kernels begin to pop.
3. Remove from heat and transfer right into a large heatproof bowl. Add essential olive oil and spices and mix well.

NUTRITION: Calories: 261 Fat: 19.45g Carbohydrates: 21.29g Protein: 2.3g

DESSERT PANCREATITIS DIET RECIPES

114.   Café-Style Fudge

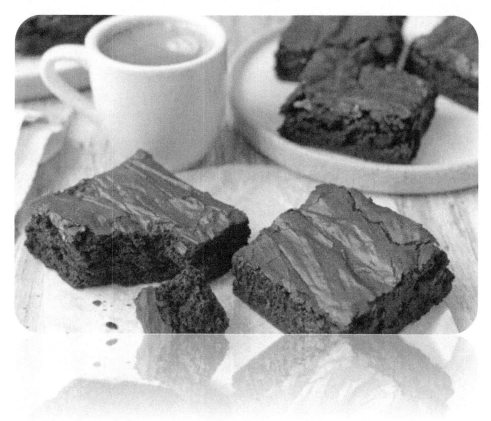

Preparation Time: 10 minutes + chilling time
Cooking time: 0 minutes
Servings: 6
INGREDIENTS:
- 1 tablespoon instant coffee granules
- 4 tablespoons confectioners' Swerve
- 4 tablespoons cocoa powder
- 1 stick butter
- 1/2 teaspoon vanilla extract

DIRECTIONS:
1. Beat the butter and Swerve at low speed. Add in the cocoa powder, instant coffee granules, and vanilla and continue to mix until well combined.
2. Spoon the batter into a foil-lined baking sheet. Refrigerate for 2 to 3 hours. Enjoy!

NUTRITION: Calories 144 Fat 15.5g Carbs 2.1g Protein 0.8g

115. Coconut and Seed Porridge

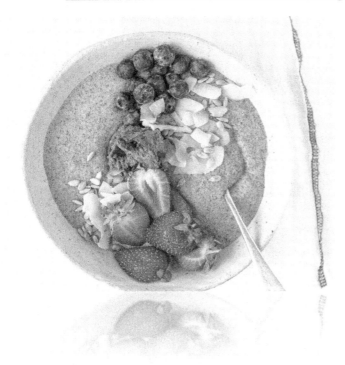

Preparation Time: 15 minutes
Cooking time: 0 minutes
Servings: 2

INGREDIENTS:

- 6 tablespoons coconut flour
- 1/2 cup canned coconut milk
- 4 tablespoons double cream
- 2 tablespoons flaxseed meal
- 1 tablespoon pumpkin seeds, ground

DIRECTIONS:

1. In a saucepan, simmer all of the above the ingredients over medium-low heat. Add in a keto sweetener of choice.
2. Divide the porridge between bowls and enjoy!

NUTRITION: Calories 300 Fat 25.1g Carbs 8g Protein 4.9g

116. Pecan and Lime Cheesecake

Preparation Time: 30 minutes + chilling time
Cooking time: 0 minutes
Servings: 10

INGREDIENTS:

- 1 cup coconut flakes

- 20 ounces mascarpone cheese, room temperature
- 1 ½ cups pecan meal
- 1/2 cup xylitol
- 3 tablespoons key lime juice

DIRECTIONS:
1. Combine the pecan meal, 1/4 cup of xylitol, and coconut flakes in a mixing bowl. Press the crust into a parchment-lined springform pan. Freeze for 30 minutes.
2. Now, beat the mascarpone cheese with 1/4 cup of xylitol with an electric mixer. Beat in the key lime juice; you can add vanilla extract, if desired.
3. Spoon the filling onto the prepared crust. Allow it to cool in your refrigerator for about 3 hours. Bon appétit!

NUTRITION: Calories 296 Fat 20g Carbs 6g Protein 21g

117.   Rum Butter Cookies

Preparation Time: 10 minutes + chilling time
Cooking time: 0 minutes
Servings: 12

INGREDIENTS:
- 1/2 cup coconut butter
- 1 teaspoon rum extract
- 4 cups almond meal
- 1 stick butter
- 1/2 cup confectioners' Swerve

DIRECTIONS:
1. Melt the coconut butter and butter. Stir in the Swerve and rum extract. Afterwards, add in the almond meal and mix to combine.
2. Roll the balls and place them on a parchment-lined cookie sheet. Place in your refrigerator until ready to serve.

NUTRITION: Calories 400 Fat 40g Carbs 4.9g Protein 5.4g

118.   Fluffy Chocolate Chip Cookies

Preparation Time: 10 minutes + chilling time
Cooking time: 0 minutes
Servings: 10

INGREDIENTS:
- 1/2 cup almond meal
- 4 tablespoons double cream
- 1/2 cup sugar-free chocolate chips
- 2 cups coconut, unsweetened and shredded
- 1/2 cup monk fruit syrup

DIRECTIONS:

1. In a mixing bowl, combine all of the above ingredients until well combined. Shape the batter into bite-sized balls.
2. Flatten the balls using a fork or your hand. Place in your refrigerator until ready to serve.

NUTRITION: Calories 104 Fat 9.5g Carbs 4.1g Protein 2.1g

119. Chewy Almond Blondies

Preparation Time: 55 minutes
Cooking time: 0 minutes
Servings: 10

INGREDIENTS:

- 1/2 cup sugar-free bakers' chocolate, chopped into small chunks
- 1/4 cup erythritol
- 2 tablespoons coconut oil
- 1 cup almond meal
- 1 cup almond butter

DIRECTIONS:

1. In a mixing bowl, combine almond meal, almond butter, and erythritol until creamy and uniform.
2. Press the mixture into a foil-lined baking sheet. Freeze for 30 to 35 minutes.
3. Melt the coconut oil and bakers' chocolate to make the glaze. Spread the glaze over your cake; freeze until the chocolate is set. Slice into bars and devour!

NUTRITION: Calories 234 Fat 25.1g Carbs 3.6g Protein 1.7g

120. Light Greek Cheesecake

Preparation Time: 15 minutes
Cooking time: 35 minutes
Servings: 6

INGREDIENTS:

- 10 ounces whipped Greek yogurt cream cheese
- 6 tablespoons butter, melted
- 2 cups confectioner's Swerve
- 2 eggs
- 2 cups almond meal

DIRECTIONS:

1. Start by preheating your oven to 325 degrees F. Combine the almond meal and butter and press the crust into a lightly buttered springform pan.
2. Beat the Greek-style yogurt with confectioner's Swerve until everything is well mixed. Fold in the eggs, one at the time, and mix well to make sure that everything is being combined together.
3. Pour the filling over the crust. Bake in the preheated oven for about 35 minutes until the middle is still jiggly. Your cheesecake will continue to set as it cools. Bon appétit!

NUTRITION: Calories 471 Fat 45g Carbs 6.9g Protein 11.5g

121.   Fluffy Chocolate Crepes

Preparation Time: 20 minutes
Cooking time: 8 minutes
Servings: 2

INGREDIENTS:

- 1/4 cup coconut milk, unsweetened
- 2 eggs, beaten
- 1/2 cup coconut flour
- 1 tablespoon unsweetened cocoa powder
- 2 tablespoons coconut oil, melted

DIRECTIONS:

1. In a mixing bowl, thoroughly combine the coconut flour and cocoa powder along with 1/2 teaspoon of baking soda.
2. In another bowl, whisk the eggs and coconut milk. Add the flour mixture to the egg mixture; mix to combine well.
3. In a frying pan, preheat 1 tablespoon of the coconut oil until sizzling. Ladle 1/2 of the batter into the frying pan and cook for 2 to 3 minutes on each side.
4. Melt the remaining tablespoon of coconut oil and fry another crepe for about 5 minutes. Serve with your favorite keto filling. Bon appétit!

NUTRITION: Calories 330 Fat 31.9g Carbs 7.1g Protein 7.3g

122.   Crispy Peanut Fudge Squares

Preparation Time: 1 hour
Cooking time: 0 minutes
Servings: 10

INGREDIENTS:

- 1/2 cup peanuts, toasted and coarsely chopped
- 1 vanilla paste
- 2 tablespoons Monk fruit powder
- 1 stick butter
- 1/3 cup coconut oil

DIRECTIONS:

1. Melt the butter, coconut oil, and vanilla. Add in Monk fruit powder and mix to combine well.
2. Place the chopped peanuts in an ice cube tray. Pour the batter over the peanuts. Place in your freezer for about 1 hour. Bon appétit!

NUTRITION: Calories 218 Fat 21.2g Carbs 5.1g Protein 3.8g

123. Almond Butter Cookies

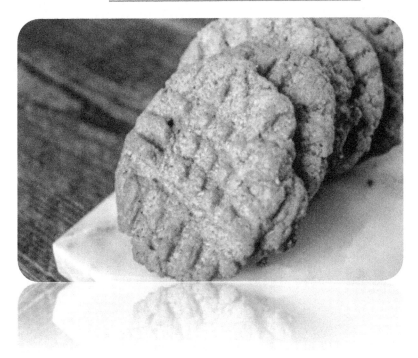

Preparation Time: 15 minutes + chilling time
Cooking time: 5 minutes
Servings: 8

INGREDIENTS:

- 1 ½ cups almond butter
- 1/2 cup sugar-free chocolate, cut into chunks
- 1/2 cup double cream
- 1/2 cup Monk fruit powder
- 3 cups pork rinds, crushed

DIRECTIONS:

1. Melt almond butter and Monk fruit powder; add in crushed pork rinds along with vanilla, if desired.
2. Spread the mixture onto a cookie sheet and place in your refrigerator.
3. Microwave the chocolate with double cream; spread the chocolate layer over the first layer. Place in your refrigerator until ready to serve. Enjoy!

NUTRITION: Calories 322 Fat 28.9g Carbs 3.4g Protein 13.9g

124. Basic Almond Cupcakes

Preparation Time: 15 minutes
Cooking time: 18-20 minutes

Servings: 9

INGREDIENTS:

- 1 cup almond milk, unsweetened
- 2 tablespoons coconut oil
- 1/2 cup almond meal
- 1/4 cup Swerve
- 3 eggs

DIRECTIONS:

1. Mix all of the above ingredients until well combined. Line a muffin pan with cupcake liners.
2. Spoon the batter into the muffin pan.
3. Bake in the preheated oven at 350 degrees F for 18 to 20 minutes or until a toothpick comes out dry and clean. Enjoy!

NUTRITION: Calories 134 Fat 11.6g Carbs 2.9g Protein 5.4g

125.   Blueberry Cheesecake Bowl

Preparation Time: 10 minutes + chilling time
Cooking time: 0 minutes
Servings: 8

INGREDIENTS:

- 2 cups cream cheese
- 1/2 cup blueberries
- 1/2 teaspoon coconut extract
- 6 tablespoons pecans, chopped
- 1/4 cup coconut cream

DIRECTIONS:

1. Beat the cream cheese and coconut cream until well mixed.
2. Fold in the coconut extract, pecans, and 1/4 cup of blueberries and mix again. Refrigerate for 2 to 3 hours. Serve garnished with the remaining 1/4 cup of blueberries. Enjoy!

NUTRITION: Calories 244 Fat 24.2g Carbs 4.7g Protein 3.7g

126.   Cacao Berry Smoothie

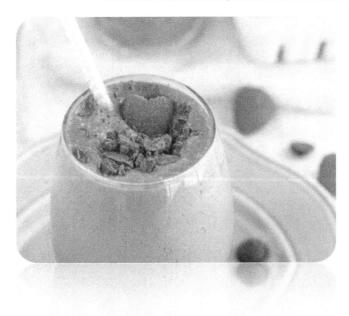

Preparation Time: 5 minutes

Cooking time: 0 minutes

Servings: 1

INGREDIENTS:

- 1 cup almond milk
- 1 banana
- 1 cup fresh baby spinach
- ½ cup filtered water
- 1 cup raspberries
- 1 tbsp. honey
- 3 tbsp. cacao powder
- ice
- cacao nibs

DIRECTIONS:

1. In a blender, combine all ingredients and mix until smooth. As desired, garnish the smoothie with cocoa nibs. Take a drink and relax.

NUTRITION: Calories: 170 Carbs: 27g Fat: 3g Protein: 5g

127.   Greek Yogurt Smoothie

Preparation Time: 5 minutes
Cooking time: 0 minutes
Servings: 1
INGREDIENTS:
- 1 cup almond milk
- ¼ cup baby spinach
- ½ cup plain Greek yogurt
- ¼ cup blueberries
- pinch of ground cinnamon
- 1 tbsp. almond butter
- cardamom
- pistachios
- 3-4 ice cubes

DIRECTIONS:
1. In a blender, combine all ingredients and pulse until smooth.

NUTRITION: Calories: 392 Carbs: 57g Fat: 10g Protein: 25g

128.   Pineapple Smoothie

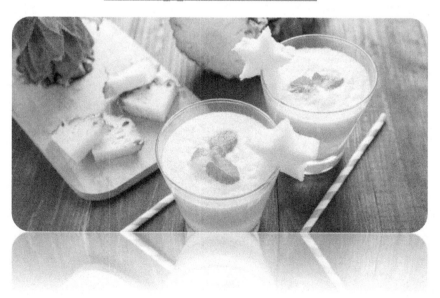

Preparation Time: 5 minutes
Cooking time: 0 minutes
Servings: 1
INGREDIENTS:
- 1 cup brewed green tea
- 1 cup frozen pineapple chunks

- 2 cups spinach
- ½ cup frozen mango chunks
- 2/3 cup cucumber
- ½ of a medium banana
- ¼ tsp. ground turmeric
- 1/2" fresh ginger
- 3 mint leaves
- 1 tbsp. chia seeds
- 1 scoop protein powder
- 4–5 ice cubes

DIRECTIONS:
1. In a high-powered blender, combine all of the ingredients, excluding the chia seeds.
2. Chia seeds should be added at the ending of the blending process to avoid sticking to the blender container.
3. If you like a thicker smoothie, add ice cubes and mix until the desired consistency is achieved.

NUTRITION: Calories: 331 Carbs: 77g Fat: 4g Protein: 0g

129.   Blueberry Banana Smoothie

Preparation Time: 5 minutes
Cooking time: 0 minutes
Servings: 2

INGREDIENTS:
- 2 cups frozen banana chunks
- 1 tsp. almond butter
- 1 cup frozen blueberries
- 1 tsp. ground flax seed
- 1¼ cups almond milk

DIRECTIONS:
1. Blend frozen blueberries, frozen banana, ground flax seed, almond butter, and almond milk until smooth in a high-powered blender.
2. Pour the smoothie into glasses and serve right away.

NUTRITION: Calories: 175 Carbs: 40g Fat: 6g Protein: 4g

130.   Blueberry Pie Smoothie

Preparation Time: 5 minutes
Cooking time: 0 minutes
Servings: 3

INGREDIENTS:
- 1 cup plain Greek yogurt
- 1 cup frozen banana chunks

- ¾ tsp. lemon zest
- ½ cup rolled oats
- 3 cups frozen blueberries
- 1½ cups almond milk
- 1/8 cup pure maple syrup
- ½ tsp. cinnamon

DIRECTIONS:
1. Blend all of the ingredients in a high-powered blender until smooth.

Nutrition: Calories: 400 Carbs: 36g Fat: 12g Protein: 28g

131.   Strawberry Banana Smoothie

Preparation Time: 5 minutes
Cooking time: 0 minutes
Servings: 3

INGREDIENTS:
- 4 cups frozen strawberries
- 1 cup milk of choice
- 1 cup frozen banana chunks

DIRECTIONS:
1. Fill your high-powered blender partially with milk.
2. On top of the milk, scatter strawberries and frozen bananas.
3. Blend on high speed until completely smooth.

NUTRITION: Calories: 120 Carbs: 29g Fat: 0g Protein: 1g

132.   Mango Pineapple Smoothie

Preparation Time: 5 minutes
Cooking time: 0 minutes
Servings: 1

INGREDIENTS:
- ½ cup frozen mango chunks
- ¾ cup almond milk
- 1 clementine, peeled
- 1 tsp. ground flax seed
- ½ cup frozen pineapple chunks
- ½ cup frozen banana chunks

DIRECTIONS:
1. Blend all of the ingredients in a high-powered blender until smooth.
2. Serve right away.

NUTRITION: Calories: 245 Carbs: 44g Fat: 2g Protein: 6g

133.   Avocado Smoothie

Preparation Time: 5 minutes
Cooking time: 0 minutes
Servings: 1
INGREDIENTS:

- 1 avocado
- 1 cup frozen pineapple
- 2 tsp. honey
- 1/3 cup vanilla Greek yogurt
- ½ cup almond milk
- 1 - 2 cups of ice

DIRECTIONS:

1. In a high-powered blender, combine all ingredients except the ice and mix until smooth.
2. Blend in the ice until it reaches the required consistency. Enjoy.

NUTRITION: Calories: 71 Carbs: 3g Fat: 6g Protein: 1g

134.   Strawberry Smoothie

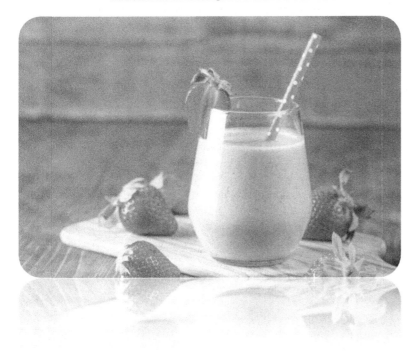

Preparation Time: 5 minutes
Cooking time: 0 minutes
Servings: 3
INGREDIENTS:

- 2 lbs. fresh strawberries

- ¼ cup milk
- 1 cup plain Greek yogurt
- 1/3 cup rolled oats
- 1/3 cup frozen pineapple
- 2 - 3 cups ice

DIRECTIONS:

1. In a blender, combine all of the ingredients and mix until smooth.
2. To get the required consistency, add more or less ice.

NUTRITION: Calories: 375 Carbs: 84g Fat: 2g Protein: 1g

135.   Beet Smoothie

Preparation Time: 5 minutes
Cooking time: 0 minutes
Servings: 1

INGREDIENTS:

- 1 small beet
- 1 ½ cups frozen mixed berries
- 1 apple
- ¼ cup plain Greek yogurt
- 2/3 cup almond milk
- 1 tsp. honey

DIRECTIONS:

1. Blend all of the ingredients in a high-powered blender until smooth.
2. Serve right away and enjoy.

NUTRITION: Calories: 205 Carbs: 0g Fat: 2g Protein: 4g

136.   Turmeric Smoothie

Preparation Time: 5 minutes
Cooking time: 0 minutes
Servings: 1

INGREDIENTS:

- 1 tsp. turmeric paste
- 1 cup frozen pineapple
- 1½ cups cold water
- 1 tsp. coconut oil
- 1 cup frozen mango
- 1 tsp. fresh ginger

DIRECTIONS:

1. In a blender, combine all of the ingredients.
2. Blend on high until completely smooth. Enjoy.

NUTRITION: Calories: 323 Carbs: 44g Fat: 18g Protein: 3g

137.   Spinach Smoothie

Preparation Time: 5 minutes
Cooking time: 0 minutes
Servings: 2

INGREDIENTS:

- 2 cups fresh spinach
- 1 large orange
- 1 cup almond milk
- 1 large banana
- 2 tbsp. ground flaxseed meal
- ice

DIRECTIONS:

1. In a large blender, combine all of ingredients and mix on high till smooth and creamy.
2. Enjoy.

NUTRITION: Calories: 316 Carbs: 52g Fat: 6g Protein: 21g

138.   Mint Chocolate Chip Smoothie

Preparation Time: 5 minutes
Cooking time: 0 minutes
Servings: 2

INGREDIENTS:

- 2 medium frozen bananas
- ¼ cup fresh mint leaves
- 1 cup almond milk
- ¼ cup chocolate chips

DIRECTIONS:

1. In a blender, combine all of the ingredients and mix until smooth.

NUTRITION: Calories: 140 Carbs: 42g Fat: 22g Protein: 17g

139.   Chocolate Protein Smoothie

Preparation Time: 5 minutes
Cooking time: 0 minutes
Servings: 1

INGREDIENTS:

- 1 ½ cups frozen strawberries
- 3 tbsp. fruit sweetener
- 1½ cups almond milk
- 3 tbsp. raw cacao powder

- 2 scoops unflavored protein

DIRECTIONS:

1. In a strong blender, combine all of the ingredients and mix until smooth.

NUTRITION: Calories: 210 Carbs: 19g Fat: 5g Protein: 24g

140.   Peach Kiwi Green Smoothie

Preparation Time: 5 minutes

Cooking time: 0 minutes

Servings: 1

INGREDIENTS:

- ¼ cup coconut milk
- 1 handful spinach leaves
- 1 kiwi, peeled
- 1 large, ripe banana
- 10 slices frozen peaches

DIRECTIONS:

1. Blend together the banana, peach slices, and coconut milk, kiwi, and spinach leaves until smooth.
2. If it's too thick, thin it out with a little almond milk until it's the right consistency.

NUTRITION: Calories: 48 Carbs: 12g Fat: 0g Protein: 0g

141.   Savory Herbed Quinoa

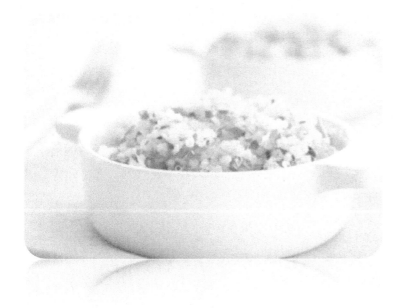

Preparation Time: 10 minutes
Cooking time: 20 minutes
Servings: 3 ½ cups

INGREDIENTS:

- 1 cup quinoa, rinsed
- 2 cups vegetable broth
- 1½ tablespoons olive oil
- Juice of ½ lemon
- ½ teaspoon salt
- ½ teaspoon freshly ground black pepper
- ½ cup chopped fresh parsley
- ½ cup chopped fresh basil
- 2 scallions, chopped

DIRECTIONS:

1. In a saucepan, combine the quinoa and broth and bring to a boil over high heat. Reduce the heat to medium-low, cover, and simmer for 15 to 20 minutes, or until the liquid is absorbed and the quinoa looks fluffy.

2. Remove from the heat and let rest, covered, for 10 minutes more. Transfer the cooked quinoa to a large bowl and add the olive oil, lemon juice, salt, pepper, parsley, basil, and scallions. Stir to incorporate.

NUTRITION: Calories: 175 Fat: 6g Protein: 5g Carbs: 25g

142. Honey-Lime Vinaigrette with Fresh Herbs

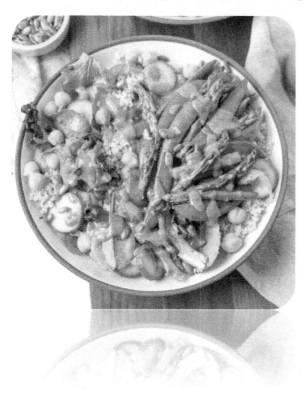

Preparation Time: 10 minutes
Cooking time: 0 minutes
Servings: 1 cup

INGREDIENTS:

- Juice of 4 limes
- 3 tablespoons honey
- 2 tablespoons apple cider vinegar
- 2 tablespoons Dijon mustard
- 2 garlic cloves, minced
- 3 scallions, finely chopped
- ½ cup roughly chopped fresh cilantro

DIRECTIONS:

1. In a medium bowl, whisk together the lime juice, honey, vinegar, mustard, and garlic. Add the scallions and cilantro and stir to combine.

NUTRITION: Calories: 82 Fat: 1g Protein: 1g Carbs: 21g

143.   Creamy Avocado Dressing

Preparation Time: 10 minutes
Cooking time: 0 minutes
Servings: 1 cup

INGREDIENTS:

- 1 avocado, halved and pitted
- 1 tablespoon olive oil
- 2 teaspoons apple cider vinegar
- 1 garlic clove, peeled but whole
- Juice of 1 lemon
- ½ teaspoon onion powder
- 1 teaspoon maple syrup
- 1 teaspoon Dijon mustard
- ½ teaspoon salt
- ½ teaspoon freshly ground black pepper
- 10 tablespoons cold water

DIRECTIONS:

1. Scoop the avocado into a food processor or blender. Add the oil, vinegar, garlic, lemon juice, onion powder, maple syrup, mustard, salt, and pepper and pulse the mixture until it's smooth and creamy.
2. Add as much water as you need, 1 tablespoon at a time, to thin it to a thick but pourable consistency.

NUTRITION: Calories: 105 Fat: 9g Protein: 1g Carbs: 7g

144.   Avocado Crema

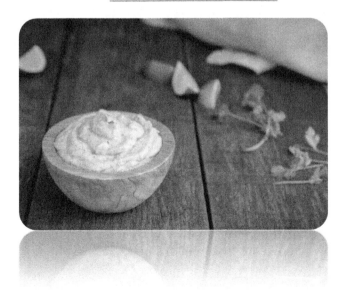

Preparation Time: 5 minutes
Cooking time: 0 minutes
Servings: 1 cup
INGREDIENTS:

- 1 avocado, halved and pitted
- ¼ cup full-fat coconut milk
- Juice of 1 lime
- ¼ teaspoon salt
- ¼ cup fresh cilantro leaves

DIRECTIONS:

1. Scoop the avocado into a food processor or blender. Add the coconut milk, lime juice, salt, and cilantro and pulse the mixture until it's smooth and creamy but still thick in consistency.

NUTRITION: Calories: 122 Fat: 11g Protein: 2g Carbs: 7g

145. Romesco

Preparation Time: 25 minutes
Cooking time: 45 minutes
Servings: 2 cups
INGREDIENTS:

- 4 red bell peppers
- 5 tablespoons extra-virgin olive oil
- Kosher salt, to taste
- ¼ cup slivered almonds
- 2 garlic cloves, peeled and coarsely chopped
- 1 shallot, sliced
- ¼ teaspoon crushed red pepper
- 1 tablespoon sherry vinegar
- Freshly ground black pepper
- 2 tablespoons chopped mint
- ½ lemon

DIRECTIONS:

1. Place a rack in the top third of the oven and preheat the oven to 400°F (205°C). Line a baking sheet with parchment paper. Place the bell peppers in a medium bowl.
2. Drizzle with 1 tablespoon of the olive oil, sprinkle with a generous pinch of salt, and toss until the peppers are well coated. Transfer to the prepared baking sheet.
3. Roast for 15 minutes, turn the peppers, and continue roasting until the peppers are charred and soft, with their skins beginning to peel away, an additional 20 minutes.
4. Transfer the peppers to a large bowl, cover tightly with plastic wrap, and let sit for 10 minutes.
5. When the peppers are cool enough to handle, remove the stems, skin, and seeds. Cut the flesh into rough strips and set aside.
6. In a medium skillet over medium heat, cook the almonds, stirring constantly, until they begin to look and smell toasted, about 4 minutes. Place them on a plate to cool.

7. Add 2 tablespoons of the olive oil to the same pan, then add the garlic, shallot, and crushed red pepper. Cook, stirring constantly, until the garlic just begins to cook and the shallot softens, about 2 minutes.
8. Place the roasted peppers and sautéed garlic and shallot in the bowl of a food processor. Pulse a few times, then add the toasted almonds.
9. Pulse a few more times, scraping down the sides of the bowl with a spatula if necessary, then add the remaining 2 tablespoons olive oil, the sherry vinegar, ¼ teaspoon salt, and a few grinds of pepper.
10. Process until the romesco is uniformly puréed but retains some texture, similar to a pesto sauce. Transfer to a small airtight container.
11. Stir in the mint, a squeeze of lemon juice, and a few grinds of pepper. Taste and season with additional salt and pepper if desired.

NUTRITION: Calories: 210 Fat: 20g Protein: 2g Carbs: 6g

146.   Creamy Turmeric Dressing

Preparation Time: 15 minutes
Cooking time: 0 minutes
Servings: 4-6
INGREDIENTS:
- ¼ cup extra-virgin olive oil
- 2 tablespoons water
- 2 tablespoons freshly squeezed lemon juice
- 1½ tablespoons raw honey
- 1 tablespoon apple cider vinegar
- 1 teaspoon ground turmeric
- 1 teaspoon Dijon mustard
- ½ teaspoon ground ginger
- ¼ teaspoon sea salt
- Pinch freshly ground black pepper

DIRECTIONS:
1. In a small bowl, combine the olive oil, water, lemon juice, honey, vinegar, turmeric, mustard, ginger, salt, and pepper. Whisk well to combine.

NUTRITION: Calories: 151 Fat: 14g Protein: 0g Carbs: 8g

147.   Cherry-Peach Chutney with Mint

Preparation Time: 15 minutes
Cooking time: 0 minutes
Servings: 2 cups
INGREDIENTS:
- 1 (10-ounce / 283-g) bag frozen no-added-sugar peach chunks, thawed, drained, coarsely chopped, juice reserved

- ½ medium red onion, diced
- ¼ cup dried cherries, coarsely chopped
- 2 tablespoons freshly squeezed lemon juice
- 1 tablespoon raw honey or maple syrup
- 1 teaspoon apple cider vinegar
- ¼ teaspoon salt
- 1 tablespoon chopped fresh mint leaves

DIRECTIONS:
1. Place the peach chunks in a medium bowl. Stir in the onion, cherries, lemon juice, honey, cider vinegar, and salt.
2. Let the mixture stand for 30 minutes before serving. When ready to serve, stir in the mint.

NUTRITION: Calories: 42 Fat: 0g Protein: 1g Carbs: 10g

148. Tofu-Basil Sauce

Preparation Time: 10 minutes
Cooking time: 0 minutes
Servings: 2 cups
INGREDIENTS:
- 1 (12-ounce / 340-g) package silken tofu
- ½ cup chopped fresh basil
- 2 garlic cloves, lightly crushed
- ½ cup almond butter
- 1 tablespoon fresh lemon juice
- 1 teaspoon salt
- ¼ teaspoon freshly ground black pepper

DIRECTIONS:
1. In a blender or food processor, combine the tofu, basil, garlic, almond butter, lemon juice, salt, and pepper. Process until smooth. If too thick, thin with a bit of water.

NUTRITION: Calories: 120 Fat: 10g Protein: 6g Carbs: 5g

149. Creamy Sesame Dressing

Preparation Time: 5 minutes
Cooking time: 0 minutes
Servings: ¾ cup
INGREDIENTS:
- ½ cup canned full-fat coconut milk
- 2 tablespoons tahini
- 2 tablespoons freshly squeezed lime juice
- 1 teaspoon bottled minced garlic
- 1 teaspoon minced fresh chives

- Pinch sea salt

DIRECTIONS:

1. In a small bowl, whisk the coconut milk, tahini, lime juice, garlic, and chives until well blended. You can also prepare this in a blender.
2. Season with sea salt and transfer the dressing to a container with a lid.

NUTRITION: Calories: 40 Fat: 4g Protein: 1g Carbs: 2g

150.   Almond-Hazelnut Milk

Preparation Time: 15 minutes
Cooking time: 0 minutes
Servings: 4 cups

INGREDIENTS:

- ½ cup-soaked raw hazelnuts, drained
- ½ cup-soaked raw almonds, drained
- 4 cups filtered water
- 1 teaspoon raw honey (optional)
- ¼ teaspoon vanilla extract (optional)

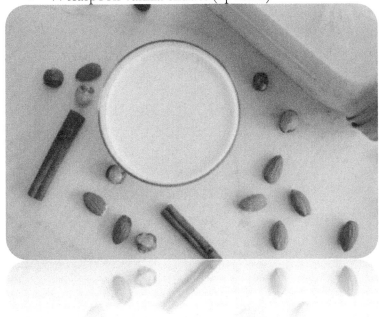

DIRECTIONS:

1. In a colander, combine the hazelnuts and almonds and give them a good rinse. Transfer to a blender and add the water. Blend at high speed for 30 seconds. 2
2. Place a nut milk bag or other mesh-like material over a large bowl and carefully pour the nut mixture into it.
3. Pick up the top of the bag and strain the liquid into the bowl, squeezing the pulp to remove as much liquid as possible.

4. Using a funnel, transfer the nut milk to a sealable bottle. Add the honey (if using) and vanilla (if using). Seal the bottle and shake well.

NUTRITION: Calories: 85 Fat: 5g Protein: 2g Carbs: 10g

28-DAY MEAL PLAN

DAY	BREAKFAST	LUNCH	DINNER	DESSERTS/SMOOTHIES
1	Salmon & Cucumber Toast	Vegan Baked Navy Bean	Beef & Sweet Potato Enchilada Casserole	Café-Style Fudge
2	Sweet Potato Omelet Pie	Grilled Salmon With Fruit And Sesame Vinaigrette	Grilled Chicken with Salad Wrap	Blueberry Cheesecake Bowl
3	Greek Yogurt with Fig Mulberries Pumpkin Seed	Tuna Au Poivre Fish Stew	Delicious Chicken Tikka Skewers	Basic Almond Cupcakes
4	Muesli Breakfast Bowl with Berries	Jalapeno Popper Chicken	Hot Lemon Prawns	Almond Butter Cookies
5	Kale & Quinoa Breakfast Bowl	Taco Stuffing	Ginger Chicken with Veggies	Crispy Peanut Fudge Squares
6	Fluffy Pancakes	Seasoned Pork Chops	Tilapia with Mushroom Sauce	Fluffy Chocolate Crepes
7	Asparagus & Tomato Omelet	Parsley Burger	Delicious Low Fat Chicken Curry	Rum Butter Cookies
8	Scramble Egg Whites Wrap	Chicken Salad Delight	Grilled Chicken Breast with Non-Fat Yogurt	Light Greek Cheesecake
9	Quick & Easy Shakshuka	Veggie "Fried" Quinoa	Peppered Steak with Cherry Tomatoes	Chewy Almond Blondies
10	Oat Pudding with	Herbed Harvest	Vegetable	Fluffy Chocolate Chip

	Chia Seeds	Rice	Tabbouleh	Cookies
11	Zucchini & Chickpeas Frittata	Coco-Nutty Brown Rice	Seared Lemon Steak with Vegetables Stir-Fry	Coconut and Seed Porridge
12	Overnight Oat Pudding Jar	Mediterranean Quinoa With Pepperoncini	Asparagus Quinoa & Steak Bowl	Pecan and Lime Cheesecake
13	Spinach & Quinoa Muffins	Indian Butter Chickpeas	Delicious Buckwheat with Mushrooms & Green Onions	Cacao Berry Smoothie
14	Cinnamon Glazed Waffle Rolls	Hatch Chile "Refried" Beans	Healthy Fried Brown Rice with Peas & Prawns	Peach Kiwi Green Smoothie
15	Pancakes Wraps	Vegan Baked Navy Bean	Yummy Chicken and Sweet Potato Stew	Chocolate Protein Smoothie
16	Salmon & Cucumber Toast	Grilled Salmon With Fruit And Sesame Vinaigrette	Slow Cooked Pork Tenderloin	Mint Chocolate Chip Smoothie
17	Sweet Potato Omelet Pie	Tuna Au Poivre Fish Stew	Herbed Salmon with Onions	Spinach Smoothie
18	Greek Yogurt with Fig Mulberries Pumpkin Seed	Jalapeno Popper Chicken	Pork with Carrots & Apples	Avocado Smoothie
19	Muesli Breakfast Bowl with Berries	Taco Stuffing	Scallop and Strawberry Salad	Turmeric Smoothie
20	Kale & Quinoa Breakfast Bowl	Seasoned Pork Chops	Easy Baked Cod	Beet Smoothie

21	Fluffy Pancakes	Parsley Burger	Pork Ragu with Tagliatelle	Strawberry Smoothie
22	Asparagus & Tomato Omelet	Chicken Salad Delight	Cilantro Halibut with Coconut Milk	Greek Yogurt Smoothies
23	Scramble Egg Whites Wrap	Veggie "Fried" Quinoa	Native Asian Soup with Squash and Shitake	Mango Pineapple Smoothie
24	Quick & Easy Shakshuka	Herbed Harvest Rice	Shredded Pork Tacos	Strawberry Banana Smoothie
25	Oat Pudding with Chia Seeds	Coco-Nutty Brown Rice	Poached Cod and Leeks	Blueberry Pie Smoothie
26	Zucchini & Chickpeas Frittata	Mediterranean Quinoa With Pepperoncini	Peppery Soup with Tomato	Pineapple Smoothie
27	Overnight Oat Pudding Jar	Indian Butter Chickpeas	Pork with Olives & Feta	Blueberry Banana Smoothie
28	Spinach & Quinoa Muffins	Hatch Chile "Refried" Beans	Halibut with Fruit Salad	Café-Style Fudge

CONCLUSION

Pancreatitis is a painful and dangerous disease that taxes the body with digestive enzymes. Treatment can include drugs, dietary changes, and surgery. It is vital to focus to nutrition while on a pancreatitis diet.

Sugar-containing foods must be limited or avoided as much as possible. As mentioned above, sugar slows down liver function by dumping an overload of sugar into your system, which the pancreas has to work harder digesting than it was designed for in the first place.

Cooked fish and meat can be added to the diet. Cod, tuna, flounder, or any other uncooked form of these foods that you find in the market are highly recommended. The reason is that they are easier to digest, and will not put a strain on your pancreas.

Soft meat in a stew or casserole form is also recommended. Cooking it in this manner will make it easier to digest and will be more slowly released into your digestive system. This is especially helpful if you find it hard to digest even cooked fish and meats.

Add soy products to your diet. This is a great source for digesting fats, proteins, and carbohydrates into your system. Soybeans are nuts in a pod, but they are gluten-free and will pick up the slack regarding protein better than any other kind of food. They can be made into anything from soups to bars and frozen desserts in order to make them more palatable to you. Just make sure that you purchase the non-gmo or organic kinds when you shop for them as well as any other food products that could be genetically modified.

Disconnect from atmospheres that pertain to unhealthy food. If you live in an environment where everyone else seems to eat, or if we eat in a certain area of the house, you might want to take a break from being around those kinds of environments. The reason is that you will be tempted to go back to eating unhealthy food rather than the best food for your pancreas.

Fiber-filled fruits and vegetables are also a necessity of the diet for pancreatitis. If you don't want fibrous vegetables such as celery and carrots, try combining them with some kind of fruit to mask the taste. It will still supply the same amount of fiber, but the taste will be more bearable for you. Make sure that you eat both these types of food at least three times per day.

Stay away from processed food, even if they're fresh and say they are healthy. They may be healthy for some people but they're not good for everyone with pancreatitis. You should avoid all dairy products even though they are delicious and nutritious proteins because they are hard on the pancreas to digest.

Sweeten anything that you consider to be sour with a natural sweetener such as honey, not corn syrup or white sugar. These are bad for your pancreas in more ways than one. These kinds of sweeteners will not actually break down in your digestive system, and will eventually cause problems. This is especially true if you have diabetes, which is a pancreas disease. The reason is that sugar can feed the candida fungus that creates all kinds of digestive problems when it grows out of control.

No more than three days of little to no carbohydrates will help with pancreatitis. Adding a low carbohydrate diet to your daily regimen will help the pancreas because it won't have to work so hard to digest the food. You must also keep all of your meal times at a maximum of 1 hour. After that, you should wait at least an hour before eating another meal again.

Keep your diet low sodium and low protein so that the pancreas doesn't have to work so hard to break down the food you eat. While you may love your salt, the excess sodium will dehydrate your pancreas and make it work harder than it needs to.

Reduce your stress levels and perform something that relaxes you. If you don't have a hobby, then take up something that you enjoy doing. You can also try going for walks in natural areas or taking a yoga class to help relax your mind and body. Whatever that works for you, do it on a regular basis as part of your healthy and daily routine while battling pancreatitis.

Never leave your meal tastebuds wanting food. I know it's tough but make yourself do it. You'll thank yourself later for not upsetting your pancreas over food. If you must have a snack, try snacking on fruits and veggies instead of sweets that are high in sugar. Never take anything that has caffeine in it. You may be a coffee drinker, but coffee will irritate your pancreas and damage it even more. This is especially true with caffeinated soda drinks.

Avoid soda drinks. Soda beverages of all kinds, whether they contain caffeine or not, are not good for you no matter how much you like them. Sugar and caffeine are not good for the pancreas. In fact, these two substances can cause the pancreas to get inflamed and damaged even more than it already is if your body is also suffering from pancreatitis at the same time.

The human body as made in such a way that it could take of all its vital processes such as digestion on its own without outside help. It was so efficiently designed that it could fix any problem with any of its organs without outside intervention. Unfortunately, with the evolution of what we eat from what our ancestors ate has rendered the body incapable of keeping up with all its processes without breaking down. This book explores one vital organ and what it is responsible for, what affects it and ways in which we can be able to keep it healthy. The first step is going back to the diet that was followed by our ancestors. As simple as eating healthy and natural foods. Feed your body with food that will nourish it and not make it seek.

I'm confident that you have been able to get important information on how to keep your pancreas healthy and how to manage any symptom of pancreatitis. Enjoy the recipes on our food section that have been specifically designed to help you manage and prevent symptoms of pancreatitis.

Remember to share with friends and family so we are able to help so many people who are living in the anguish of pancreatitis pain.

All the best as you embrace a healthier life that is now more informed!

RECIPE INDEX

A

Almond Butter Cookies 116

Almond-Hazelnut Milk 132

Apple Leather 108

Apricot Salad with Mustardy Dressing 55

Asparagus & Tomato Omelet 36

Asparagus Quinoa & Steak Bowl 66

Avocado Crema 128

Avocado Smoothie 122

B

Basic Almond Cupcakes 116

Beef & Sweet Potato Enchilada Casserole 63

Beet Chips 106

Beet Smoothie 123

Blueberry Banana Smoothie 120

Blueberry Cheesecake Bowl 117

Blueberry Pie Smoothie 120

Bone in Ham with Maple-Honey Glaze 83

C

Cacao Berry Smoothie 118

Café-Style Fudge 111

Carrot Salad with Lemony Cashew Dressing 58

Cherry & Apple Pork 77

Cherry-Peach Chutney with Mint 130

Chewy Almond Blondies 114

Chicken Salad Delight 47

Chili Coconut Salmon 90

Chinese Salmon 88

Chipotle Pork Carnitas 78

Chocolate Protein Smoothie 124

Cilantro Halibut with Coconut Milk 86

Cinnamon Glazed Waffle Rolls 32

Clams with Olives Mix 91

Classic Soup with Butternut Squash 93

Classic Vegetarian Tagine 98

Classy Soup with Carrot and Ginger 92

Coconut and Seed Porridge 112

Coco-Nutty Brown Rice 45

Corn Chowder 101

Corned Pork 78

Crab Salad 89

Creamy Avocado Dressing 128

Creamy Sesame Dressing 131

Creamy Soup with Broccoli 93

Creamy Turmeric Dressing 130

Crispy Peanut Fudge Squares 115

Cucumber and Spinach with Chicken Salad 57

D

Delicious Buckwheat with Mushrooms & Green Onions 64

Delicious Chicken Tikka Skewers 72

Delicious Low Fat Chicken Curry 70

Delicious Pork Roast Baracoa 75

E

Easy Baked Cod 87

Egg Drop Soup 102

Extraordinary Creamy Green Soup 95

F

Fish Stew 50

Fluffy Chocolate Chip Cookies 113

Fluffy Chocolate Crepes 115

Fluffy Pancakes 37

G

Garlic Cod Soup 89

Garlicky Broccoli with Cashew Soup 59

Ginger Chicken with Veggies 71

Greek Yogurt Smoothie 119

Greek Yogurt with Fig Mulberries Pumpkin Seed............38

Grilled Chicken Breast with Non-Fat Yogurt....................69

Grilled Chicken with Salad Wrap 73

Grilled Salmon With Fruit And Sesame Vinaigrette.........51

H

Halibut with Fruit Salad 85

Hatch Chile "Refried" Beans 42

Healthy Fried Brown Rice with Peas & Prawns................65

Herbed Harvest Rice 45

Herbed Salmon with Onions...88

Homemade Warm and Chunky Chicken Soup 99

Honey-Lime Vinaigrette with Fresh Herbs 127

Hot Lemon Prawns 71

I

Indian Butter Chickpeas..43

Indian Curried Stew with Lentil and Spinach 100

J

Jalapeno Popper Chicken 49

K

Kale & Quinoa Breakfast Bowl...37

L

Lemony Zucchini with Vinegary Salmon 57

Light Greek Cheesecake.. 114

M

Mango Pineapple Smoothie 121

Mediterranean Quinoa With Pepperoncini........................44

Milky Carrot with Oniony Ginger Soup............................59

Mint Chocolate Chip Smoothie 124

Minty Melon with Vinegar 53

Mixed Greens Salad with Honeyed Dressing....................54

Mixed Greens Soup with Coconut Milk 60

Moroccan Inspired Lentil Soup...97

Muesli Breakfast Bowl With Berries.................................38

N

Native Asian Soup with Squash and Shitake 96

O

Oat Pudding with Chia Seeds..35

Okra Fries 104

Onion Chipotle Soup with Sage 61

Overnight Oat Pudding Jar 33

P

Paleo Italian Pork...77

Pancakes Wraps..31

Parsley Burger 47

Peach Kiwi Green Smoothie... 125

Pears with Peppered Fennel Soup 61

Pecan and Lime Cheesecake 112

Peppered Steak with Cherry Tomatoes..............................68

Peppery Soup with Tomato 97

Pineapple Smoothie.. 119

Plantain Chips 107

Poached Cod and Leeks 86

Pork Casserole 75

Pork Egg Roll Soup..74

Pork Ragu with Tagliatelle 81

Pork with Carrots & Apples 80

Pork with Olives & Feta 82

Potato Caraway with Lemony Fillet...................................56

Potato Sticks 105

Q

Quick & Easy Shakshuka 35

Quinoa & Seeds Crackers 108

R

Roasted Cashews 109

Roasted Pumpkin Seeds 109

Romesco 129

Rum Butter Cookies 113

S

Salmon & Cucumber Toast 30

Savory Herbed Quinoa 126

Scallion with Minty Cucumber Salad 62

Scallop and Strawberry Salad 84

Scramble Egg Whites Wrap 36

Seared Lemon Steak with Vegetables Stir-Fry 67

Seasoned Pork Chops 48

Shredded Pork Tacos 81

Slow Cooked Pork Tenderloin 80

Soulful Roasted Vegetable Soup 100

Spiced Popcorn 110

Spinach & Quinoa Muffins 33

Spinach and Scallop 88

Spinach Chips 106

Spinach Smoothie 124

Squashy Carrot and Celery Soup 60

Strawberry Banana Smoothie 121

Strawberry Smoothie 122

Swedish Meatballs & Mushrooms Gravy 76

Sweet & Tangy Seeds Crackers 107

Sweet Potato Omelet Pie 39

T

Taco Stuffing 48

Thai Soup with Potato 94

Tilapia with Mushroom Sauce 70

Tofu-Basil Sauce 131

Tuna Au Poivre 50

Turmeric Smoothie 123

V

Vegan Baked Navy Beans 41

Vegetable Tabbouleh 67

Veggie "Fried" Quinoa 46

Vinegary Berry with Orange Salad 56

Y

Yummy Chicken and Sweet Potato Stew 65

Z

Zingy Soup with Ginger, Carrot, and Lime 95

Zucchini & Chickpeas Frittata 34

Zucchini Chips 105

Made in the USA
Las Vegas, NV
07 April 2022

47036376R10079